Anti-Inflammatory Diet for Beginners

4 Week Diet Plan to Reverse Chronic Inflammation and Revitalize your Life by Losing Weight and Reducing Long-Term Disease Risks *through Simple Dietary Changes*

NICHOLAS STEPHENS

© Copyright 2019 – by Nicholas Stephens - All rights reserved.

The content contained within this book may not be reproduced, duplicated or transmitted without direct written permission from the author or the publisher.

Under no circumstances will any blame or legal responsibility be held against the publisher, or author, for any damages, reparation, or monetary loss due to the information contained within this book, either directly or indirectly.

Legal Notice:

This book is copyright protected. It is only for personal use. You cannot amend, distribute, sell, use, quote or paraphrase any part, or the content within this book, without the consent of the author or publisher.

Disclaimer Notice:

Please note the information contained within this document is for educational and entertainment purposes only. All effort has been executed to present accurate, up to date, reliable, complete information. No warranties of any kind are declared or implied. Readers acknowledge that the author is not engaging in the rendering of legal, financial, medical or professional advice. The content within this book has been derived from various sources. Please consult a licensed professional before attempting any techniques outlined in this book.

By reading this document, the reader agrees that under no circumstances is the author responsible for any losses, direct or indirect, that are incurred as a result of the use of information contained within this document, including, but not limited to, errors, omissions, or inaccuracies.

TABLE OF CONTENTS

Indice generale

Introduction..1

Chapter 1: What Is Inflammation?..6

Chapter 2: Anti-Inflammatory Diets and How They Can Improve Your Overall Health..13

Chapter 3: Preparing to Practice the Anti Inflammatory Diet...................22

Chapter 4: Week 1 Recipes...32

Chapter 5: Week 2 Recipes...65

Chapter 6: Week 3 Recipes...98

Chapter 7: Week 4 Recipes...126

Chapter 8: Snack Recipes...154

Chapter 9: Beverages...178

Conclusion..197

References...199

Introduction

Congratulations on purchasing *Anti-Inflammatory Diet for Beginners.* Leave a brief review on Amazon if you like it, I'd really love to hear what you think.

To understand why anti-inflammatory diets are so effective at wading off the risk of certain diseases and generally revitalizing your life, you first need to understand what inflammation is, why it is needed, and when it becomes dangerous.

Inflammation is a complex process and it can be of two kids: acute inflammation and chronic. Inflammation is one of the body's natural and most effective defenses against infection of pathogens such as viruses, bacteria, and injury to cells. From infancy, all people become acquainted with the symptoms of inflammation. The word 'symptoms' creates the impression of something scary, which should be avoided but inflammation is a good thing as it is a sign that your body is healing itself.

Acute inflammation occurs frequently and occurs where the body naturally heals itself through the inflammatory process. If you have ever had sprained your ankle or went in for a vaccine, you would have noticed swelling, warmth, and pain around the affected area. Be thankful that this occurred because this is the process of inflammation at work.

But what happens when the body goes haywire and does not know how to control this process? What happens when the body starts attacking itself with a process meant to protect? The answer: damage to the body.

Just like with conditions such as asthma and eczema, the body can become overzealous with its need to protect itself and thus cause more damage than good. This is the case when chronic inflammation occurs. While acute inflammation is an effective protective mechanism that the body has developed to get itself back to working at its optimal conditions as fast as possible in case of injury or infection, chronic inflammation persists over a longer period of time, often not clearing in the correct manner. This causes harm to tissues and cells, and can become so severe that medical intervention is needed, and even then there may not be much that the sufferer can do to reverse the symptoms. The problem is so severe that that chronic inflammation is a disease and has become one of the greatest contributing factors to some of today's most other common chronic diseases. Heart disease, autoimmune dysfunctions, obesity, Alzheimer's disease, and even some forms of cancer are a result of chronic inflammation.

You Can Fight the Debilitating Symptoms of Chronic Inflammation with A Few Simple Changes to Your Diet and Lifestyle

One of the most powerful weapons you can use to fight any of the diseases that are rampant in today's society is knowledge and the same is true with chronic inflammation. This book aims to provide you with the understanding of how chronic inflammation works, what causes it, and what you can do to reduce the effects if it becomes a problem in your life.

Today's society has promoted quick fixes and instant gratification for most problems. However, one cannot slap a bandage on chronic inflammation. Most drugs such as ibuprofen for pain relief only offer a short-term solution. There are even special anti-inflammatory prescription drugs offered to sufferers, but they do not take away the cause of the problem. As a result, the inflammation will persist.

Instead, chronic inflammation needs long-term and strategic solutions, and one of these is making changes to your diet and lifestyle. The reason that diet is such an important contributing factor to decreasing the problem of chronic inflammation is because many of the foods that we eat and drink everyday introduce toxins into our bodies. The body then tries to attack and eliminate these toxins by increasing the instances of inflammation. In addition to causing the flare-up of inflammation, these toxins contribute toward a number of other health problems, hence the epidemic that is widespread with an increasing number of obesity and heart disease cases, and a myriad of other health issues worldwide.

Processed food is one of the most dangerous to consume yet most people do so daily. Everyday we introduce artificial ingredients, bad carbohydrates, large amounts of sugar, and many more harmful ingredients to the body. It is no wonder that inflammation and the other associated diseases are on the rise. The convenience of these foods is clearly overshadowed by the fact that they are addictive and use the body as dumping ground for toxins.

Control Inflammation to Improve Your Overall Health

Your body is a temple. You only get one body. Therefore, you should do everything in your power to ensure that you care for it in the best way possible. General health and wellness are directly related to eating habits.

The age old saying of "You are what you eat," is as true today as it was a century ago. By taking control of what you eat, when you eat it, and how you eat it, you can control the way you look, feel, and think.

If you consume processed foods and foods high in sugar but skimp on your veggies and fruits, it will be reflected in your waistline, probably in the acne on your cheeks and even in the luster of your hair. But the problems are not limited to your physical appearance. In fact, the external signs of a poor diet are normally just a glimpse of what is going on within.

By eating clean, wholesome, and fresh foods, you can control how your body deposits fat, how it detoxes itself and the amount of detoxification it goes through, it has to do and the good nutrients it has available. The internal conditions of your body will thrive and it will reflect in the outer appearance of your body. Your will like become slimmer, have healthier skin and fuller hair. You will also improve your mental and emotional states, promoting a happier, more fulfilled you.

Most often, controlling chronic inflammation is as easy as controlling your diet. Participating in an anti inflammatory diet detoxifies the body and helps facilitate the healing process in a healthy way. The widespread benefits of practicing an anti inflammatory diet on the inflammation process and general health and wellness are not just hearsay. Medical research and studies have repeatedly shown that an anti inflammatory diet protects the body against many acute and chronic diseases including chronic inflammation. The diet does this by enhancing the metabolic processes of the body as well as stabilizing blood sugar and cholesterol levels, all processes that promote an overall healthy individual.

There are no disadvantages to practicing an anti inflammatory diet even if you do not suffer from chronic inflammation. While this book is meant to provide you with the knowledge that you need to fight chronic inflammation in a practical, actionable way, it is also meant to show you that this diet, along with other lifestyle such as a proper exercise regiment, can allow you to achieve your health goals in a painless, progressive way.

The pages to come are information-packed and founded on sound studies and sources. You will learn more on the differences between acute and chronic inflammation, how to prepare your body for an anti inflammatory diet, the foods you should eat and those you should avoid to decrease the likelihood of chronic inflammation, and those that are most effective in promoting the production of pro-inflammatory substances within the body. In addition, you will be given over 100 recipes for breakfast, lunch, dinner, and everything in between to make this a tasty journey for you as well. The included information on grocery shopping and the food pyramid depicting recommended serving sizes and nutritional values will also help you experiment and create your own recipes that do not undo the hard work you have put into reaping the rewards of this diet.

This is a guidebook and cookbook combined into one powerful source of all things inflammation! And best yet, the information has been assimilated for an easy-to-read, seamless flow using terminology that that anyone can understand.

Turn to the next page to better understand inflammation and how it affects your daily life, to change your outlook on your diet for overall wellness and to improve your diet so that your can live happier, healthier, and more holistically.

Chapter 1: What Is Inflammation?

In the introductory chapter, we supplied the basic definition what inflammation is. However, the process is more in-depth and far more complicated than the surface signs that we see. Inflammation one of the body's first lines of defense in response to injury, trauma or infection. It is a signal that the immune system needs to repair and heal damaged tissue as well as put up a line of defense against foreign entities such as bacteria and viruses. This process is facilitated by the presence of white blood cells and other substances that protect the body come foreign or outside invaders. In essence, the body unleashes a mini army to clear out any malevolent invaders. This army release is facilitated by chemical signals that tell the white blood cells aka the soldiers in this army, where to stand and when to start fighting.

In addition to all these complex advantages, inflammation also limits the area where tissue is damaged and stops the spread of foreign microbes as to minimize the damage caused. Inflammation also clears away any debris that is created from the process so that the tissue can heal in a clean and safe environment.

Without this physiological line of defense, wounds would not heal and instead they would fester. Without this defense, infections would overrun the body and become deadly. Without inflammation, the human population will dwindle down to nothing.

What Happens When Inflammation Goes on for Too Long?

There are two types of inflammation. The first is called acute inflammation it is a short-term response to the site of a problem such as a cut on the knee, burn, broken bone or scraped flesh. symptoms include:

- Pain
- Redness
- Swelling
- Heat at the site of the existing problem
- Loss of function at the site

When acute inflammation occurs, the body responds by dilating blood vessels to increase blood flow to the site of the problem. At the site of injury or infection, tissue in need of aid releases a chemical called cytokines which signal the need for white blood cells to the injured or infected area to promote healing. Nutrients are also delivered to the site to aid in the healing process.

Substances called prostaglandins are also released at the site. They promote blood clotting to heal damaged tissue and also cause pain and fever, both of which are signs that the healing process has been activated.

As the body heals, the symptoms of inflammation gradually

subside and cease altogether. Pain, redness, swelling, and the other common symptoms of inflammation stop. After cells have regenerated themselves and tissue has healed itself, the site of inflammation is restored to a normal appearance. Blood flow resumes to normal and white blood cells return to their normal levels and functions within the body.

It is not only physical injury that activates acute inflammation. Radiation, chemical irritants, and toxins also cause an instant flare-up of inflammation depending on the level of exposure and hazardousness. Infection of bacteria, viruses, and other foreign pathogens also cause inflammation although there may be a delay in the show of symptoms as the attack on the body occurs internally rather than from the outside. A common example of this is a sore throat.

To make the process of acute inflammation clearer in your mind, let's break it down into the individual steps:

1. A harmful stimulus such as a cut or pathogens are detected by the body.
2. Cells belonging to the immune system at the site of the infected tissue become active. Their receptors detected the damage or invasion. They then release chemicals that dilate blood vessels nearby to increase blood flow to the site.
3. This increased blood flow brings white blood cells to the site. Glucose, which is a sugar, and oxygen are also delivered to the site. They nourish the cells there, increasing their ability to repair and heal the damaged tissue. As a result of the blood vessel dilation, plasma proteins and antibodies are also delivered to the site.

4. Swelling, heat, pain, and redness occur at the site as a result of the above conditions and reactions. Even more white blood cells are delivered, especially if a pathogenic infection is the cause of this process activation. These cells not only destroy the pathogens, they also help repair any wounds. The presence of white blood cells also wards off any further attacks from pathogens.
5. Once the pathogens have been isolated, cleanup commences. Dead cells, both internal and invasive, and other debris created in the healing process are removed from the site. New cells replace the old ones and excess white blood cells leave the area. Once all of this is done, everything at the site returns to normal.

This a smooth process but sometimes there is a breakdown in this process, which is what occurs with the other type of inflammation.

Chronic Inflammation and Why it is Harmful

Remember the old saying that "Too much of a good thing is bad?" This saying applies in this case as well. Inflammation can go on for too long or can occur in places where it is not needed. This is what occurs in the second form of inflammation, which is called chronic inflammation. This type of inflammation is also called persistent, low-grade inflammation because it occurs over a prolonged of time unlike acute inflammation which usually persists for a few days or less. Chronic inflammation can persist for years and causes cellular destruction, scar tissue, fibrosis, and abscess formation to occur. This condition is a disease and needs to be treated at the earliest to avoid the negative consequences.

Referring to the smooth process outlined above in the case of acute inflammation, chronic inflammation often breakdowns at the termination phase of the process. In fact, the process does not stop and one reason for this is that white blood cells and other chemicals released by the immune system periodically check cells for normalities. If all is normal, then they terminate the inflammation process. With chronic inflammation, the immune system cells mistake normal body cells for harmful cells and continue attacking at the site. It destroys the cells, thus harming the body rather than curing it.

Chronic inflammation is harmful on its own but the dangers only increase as it has been linked to several diseases. Some of these common diseases are cardiovascular diseases such as stroke or heart disease and autoimmune disorders like lupus, rheumatoid arthritis, gouty arthritis, and psoriatic arthritis. Cancer is another disease that has been linked to this condition as it causes damage of DNA, thus giving rise to abnormalities. The cancers that may be a result of inflammation include colon cancer, breast cancer, and colorectal cancer.

Chronic inflammation is often characterized by symptoms such as:

- Joint pain
- Joint stiffness
- Loss of brain function
- Swollen joints that can be warm to the touch

While these listed above are the most common symptoms of chronic inflammation, some people may experience flu-like symptoms as well. These include:

- Headaches
- Chills

- Fever
- Muscle stiffness
- Loss of appetite
- Fatigue

Other unusual symptoms include chronic diarrhea and numbness to one side of the face.

What Causes Chronic Inflammation?

Inflammation can be caused by any number of physical, biological, chemical, psychological, and environmental factors. As a result of these factors, there are people who are at greater risk of developing chronic inflammation. By being informed about these, you can first evaluate yourself for these risk factors then take the appropriate steps to prevent chronic inflammation.

Those Most At Risk For Chronic Inflammation

They are:

- People who have suffered from blunt or penetrating physical injuries like frostbite and burns.
- People who are overweight or obese. This is due to the fact that the body naturally attacks fat deposits as they are mistaken for foreign entities. This causes the fat cells to break, resulting in leakages activate the inflammation process.
- People with a history of heart disease or heart disease in the family.
- People with type 2 diabetes. This is a two-fold process as people with this type of diabetes

normally develop inflammation while people with chronic inflammation typically develop type 2 diabetes.
- People who frequent toxic environments.
- People who suffer from chronic fatigue.
- People who suffer from high levels of stress or mental disorders like depression.
- Older people. This is because human beings tend to release more chemicals that promote inflammation and less of anti-inflammatory chemicals as they get older.

How is Chronic Inflammation Diagnosed?

Chronic inflammation is diagnosed by testing the blood for certain indicators. Such indicators include:

- The existence of the protein molecule called cytokine. This molecule is secreted to regulate the immune system. There are two types of cytokines and they are called tumor necrosis factor alpha (TNFa) and interleukin-6 (IL-6). IL-6 is the one to look out for as it is a proinflammatory chemical and triggers the initial phases of acute inflammation.
- High levels of CRP (C-reactive protein). CRP is produced in the liver in response to inflammation.
- Analysis through serum protein electrophoresis (SPE). This is a measure of certain proteins in blood cells. Too much and too little of these particular proteins can signal inflammation in addition to other conditions.
- Analysis of the Erythrocyte Sedimentation Rate

(ESR). This blood test measures the rate at which red blood cells sink in a tube of blood. If they sink quickly, this can be an indicator of inflammation. This taste is called a sedimentation rate test and is usually done in conjunction with other tests.
- The thickness of blood. Inflammation can cause the blood to thicken.

There are other diagnostic tests that can be done and these include:

- Colonoscopy
- Sigmoidoscopy
- Upper endoscopy

These are tests on the digestive tract.

X-rays and MRIs can also be performed to check certain parts of the body upon request by doctors.

Chapter 2: Anti-Inflammatory Diets and How They Can Improve Your Overall Health

Diets have become all the rage these days with fancy names and outrageous meal plans and unusual recipes. The anti inflammatory diet is not a fancy term nor does it require any off the wall recipes to work. In fact, I would go so far as to say that it is not even a particular diet, but a variety of other diets combined to develop a comprehensive eating plan that optimizes the way your body works.

Types of Eating Regimens to Reduce Chronic Inflammation

Mediterranean Diet

This eating regimen is inspired by the eating habits of people who live in the Mediterrean region. This eating regimen consists of a high consumption of olive oil, fruits, vegetables, legumes, and unrefined grains in addition to seafood and dairy products like cheese and yogurt. Red meats are resisted in the preparation of Mediterranean meals. There is also a great emphasis on the consumption of wine!

This eating regimen is a great addition to the anti inflammatory diet because it reduces inflammatory indicators such as IL-6 and CRP because of is beneficial injection of dietary fibers and monounsaturated fats into the diet while keeping saturated fats low.

The other health benefits of this eating regimen include lowering the rates of neurodegeneration, certain chronic diseases, cardiovascular diseases, and reducing the risk of cancer. These benefits are largely due to the use of olive oil because of its anti inflammatory benefits due to the presence of a fatty acid called oleic acid. Olive oil also contains antioxidants, which are substances that removes potentially damaging oxidizing agents from the body, helps prevent cardiovascular disease and is not associated with weight gain despite being an oil.

Vegetarian and Vegan Diets

These two eating regimens consist of principally plant-based foods which are rich in vitamin K. Dark, green, and leafy vegetables like spinach, kale, and broccoli are largely used in these two types of eating plans. They have long been known to fight the symptoms of chronic inflammation.

Fruits are also a big part of these two eating plans. Colorful fruits such as blackberries and raspberries are particularly helpful in fighting inflammation as the pigment that produces their vibrant colors contains a vital substance for fighting the symptoms.

In addition, these regimens promote the use of vegan protein sources and fish instead of red meat. Combined, all of these components aid in increasing the levels of plasma amino acid, which is an indicator of lowered risk of inflammation and by extension, heart disease.

Low Carb Eating Diet

The title is largely self-explanatory and not only does it help reduce the instances of chronic inflammation, but it also helps to reduce other health issues such as high blood pressure, diabetes, cardiovascular diseases, and many digestive issues. The principal of this eating regiment entails replacing easily digestible low-carb foods such as bread, rice, sugar, and pasta with foods that are rich in fats yet moderate in proteins. These replacements usually come in the form of seafood, nuts, and seeds, dairy, dark green leafy vegetables or fruits.

There are several low carb diets out there but some of the most effective at helping fight inflammation are the ketogenic diet, the Atkins diet, and the paleo diet all of which are based on a low carb intake.

Eating for Better Health and Anti Inflammation

Foods that Increase the Risk of Chronic Inflammation and that Should be Avoided

As a general rule of thumb, anything that is highly processed, overly sweet, greasy, and packaged can increase your risk of developing chronic inflammation. You may be tempted to reach for them when you go to the supermarket, but muster up that resistance to do so. In fact, they should be completely crossed off from your shopping list and meal plans.

To make it even easier, here is a comprehensive list of the foods that should be avoided in order to reduce the risk of developing chronic inflammation.

Red meats that have been processed and contain high fats

Example of these includes hot dogs and sausages. They contain high amounts of saturated fats, something which has been shown to directly cause inflammation.

Processed whole milk, cheese, and butter

These have a high saturated fat content. Only low-fat dairy products should be consumed.

Fried foods

While the body does need a moderate amount of fatty acids, consuming foods that have been fried in vegetable oil such as corn oil increases the amount of omega-6 fatty acids in the body. The increase in omega-6 fatty acids may disturb the amount of Omega-3 fatty acids and this imbalance gives rise to inflammatory problems.

Foods that contain trans fats

Trans fats also known as trans fatty acids are derived from solid fats which have been converted from liquid vegetable oil in a process called hydrogenation. Trans fats increase the levels of low-density lipoproteins (LDL) which is a bad cholesterol and which causes the flare-up of inflammation. Even products on your grocery shelf that carry a partially hydrogenated fat or oil in the ingredient list should be avoided even if it is just minute traces of trans fat.

Refined carbohydrates

Refined carbohydrates differ from unrefined carbohydrates in that they are process to remove a lot of the natural nutrition resulting in a loss of essential vitamins and minerals. Common refined carbohydrates include white bread and white pasta. Due to their high sugar and carbohydrate components, they cause the body to release cytokines which is an inflammatory agent. Not only do they increase the risk of chronic inflammation but they cause weight gain, high cholesterol levels, and high blood sugar conditions which are bad for overall health and wellness.

Sweetened foods and beverages

Foods that contain a high amount of sugars, such as soda, fruit juices, and sugary snacks should be avoided. Even honey and agave cause flare-ups in inflammation.

Glutinous grains

Gluten is the substance that is generated when water is mixed with water soluble proteins found in wheat and green flowers. gluten has been shown to aggravate inflammation therefore grains such as wheat, rye and barley should be avoided.

Nightshades

Nightshades are mostly comprised of plants, shrubs, and herbs that are poisonous, but some edible fruits such as potatoes and eggplant, which are safe to eat stimulate chronic inflammation.

Foods that are Good to Eat

Fruits and Vegetables

By consuming these, you stock up on the essential vitamins, minerals, and antioxidants the body needs to support the immune system and thus reduce chronic inflammation. Deeply colored fruit varieties like raspberries, grapes, oranges, blackberries, and fruits that are high in good fats like olives and avocados are the best choice. Many berries contain the antioxidant called anthocyanin, which offers anti inflammatory, antiviral and anti cancer benefits.

As for veggies, reach for the dark, green leafy types first.

These include collard greens, kale, spinach, and broccoli to name a few. Broccoli in particular is rich in sulforaphane, an antioxidant that helps reduce cytokine levels to fight inflammation.

To gain the best nutrition out of these, adults should consume up to two cups of fresh fruit three times daily and three cups of organic vegetables four times daily.

Unrefined Whole Grains

Get your essential vitamins and iron from consuming these. Not only are you benefitting from the nutritional value, but there are several other benefits such as reducing cholesterol levels through the stabilization of blood sugar levels, aiding in weight loss management by suppressing the hormones that trigger hunger signals, and it also helps circulate oxygen-rich red blood cells throughout the entire body. Consuming unrefined whole grains such as whole grain or multigrain bread that has been sweetened with fruit sweeteners such as raisins, brown rice, and unrefined cereal grains like quinoa and bulgur also help lower your risk of developing cardiovascular disease. Adults should consume unrefined whole grains four times a day.

Nuts and Seeds

Nuts like almonds, cashew nuts, peanuts, Brazil nuts, walnuts, and pistachios, and seeds like chia seeds, pumpkin seeds, and ground flaxseed contain healthy monounsaturated fats, fiber, and protein to help you lose weight and control inflammation as long as they are consumed in moderation. No more than a handful or 1.5 ounces should be consumed daily by adults. Other notable nuts include hazelnuts and pine nuts and nutritious seeds include hemp and sesame seeds.

Fatty Fish

These include tuna, sardines, herring, cod, salmon, anchovies, and mackerel. They contain omega-3 fatty acids that lower IL-6 and CRP quantities to reduce the incidence of inflammation. Fatty fish should be consumed between twice and six times a week in quantities of around 4 ounces.

Healthy Herbs and Spices

Use less salt and add flavor to your food the natural and safe way. You can stock up your spice cabinets with the following herbs and spices to not only make your food taste great but to prevent chronic inflammation:

- Ginger, which can be used in both sweet and savory dishes, contains the antioxidant gingerol, which packs quite the punch to reduce many gastrointestinal disorders and to treat the pain of rheumatoid arthritis.
- Turmeric contains a chemical called curcumin. This helps fight other conditions related to chronic inflammation such as Alzheimer's disease and arthritis. Turmeric is most effective when combined with black pepper because it is absorbed by the body better. This is what gives curry powder its vibrant color.
- Garlic contains an anti inflammatory compound that inhibits proinflammatory compounds such as cytokines. It also helps relieve pain and fights against cartilage damage caused by arthritis.
- Cinnamon has antioxidant properties. In addition to its aid in anti inflammation, it helps the body repair damage done to cells by free radicals.
- Sweet and spicy peppers help reduce

inflammation and relieve pain because they contain capsaicin compounds. Bell peppers and chilli peppers are packed with antioxidants and vitamin C, both of which promote anti inflammation.

Beans and Legumes

This food group includes red kidney beans, garbanzos, chickpeas, lentils, and black beans. They are rich in antioxidants, good fats, fiber, iron, zinc, potassium, folate, and magnesium, all of which are anti inflammatory substances. It is great to consume one cup of beans and legumes two times a day.

Soy

Soy-based foods are a great source of fiber, which help keep your digestive system in good working order. These foods should be consumed once or twice daily and include items such as tofu, soybeans, soy flour, soymilk, soy nuts, and tempeh.

Natural Teas

It is a great idea to consume natural teas such as green, black, white, and ginger about three times a day. These help protect the body from several diseases, many of which are associated with chronic inflammation. They have this power because they are steeped in polyphenols. Teas are also a great source of antioxidants, which helps fight chronic inflammation. Green tea contains a substance called EGCCG (epigallocatechin-3-gallate), which reduces cytokine levels.

Red Wine

This contains a compound called resveratrol, which is an

anti inflammatory substance. It also contains antioxidants to protect the body from certain cancers and cardiovascular disease. One of the most widely talked about benefits of red wine are its anti aging properties. When consumed in moderation that is. The recommended daily serving is five ounces or less for women and 10 ounces or less for men.

Certain Sweets

If you have a sweet tooth, do not fear. Not all sweets are banned from the anti inflammatory diet. Select sweets such as plain dark chocolate and plant-based syrups like maple syrup and fruit sugars are allowed. Dark chocolate in packed with antioxidants. Ensure that if you indulge in this sweet that it has at least 70% cocoa to enjoy the most anti inflammatory benefits.

Anti Inflammatory Supplements

Common supplements used to fight chronic inflammation include garlic, fish oils, and onions. However, you can boost the benefits of these by also taking berberine, spirulina, ALA (alpha lipoic acid), and curcumin.

Berberine is a tonic supplement. Extracted from goldenseal or barberry plants, it helps treat gastrointestinal problems such as IBS (irritable bowel syndrome) and UC (ulcerative colitis) which is inflammation of the colon, is an antibacterial agent and also helps reduce fever. This supplement also helps lower blood sugar levels.

Spirulina is a probiotic and helps promote the growth and balance of good bacteria in the gut. It is obtained from blue-green algae called cyanobacteria. This supplement is rich in vitamins A and B12 as well as some minerals and proteins. These help reduce chronic inflammation and the resulting negative effects.

ALA helps eliminate heavy metals such as mercury, lead, and copper, which can be harmful, from the bloodstream. It is an antioxidant and healthy fatty acid.

Curcumin helps reduce fever and is a natural pain reliever.

A Helpful Shopping List

It is always a good idea to keep your cabinets and refrigerator stocked with the good stuff that will help you fight inflammation rather than promote it. Below you can find anti inflammatory products that you can find at most grocery stores. These make a good compliment to the items already listed above.

Fruits

Grapefruits, bananas, cucumbers, apples, lemons, limes, mangoes, pomegranates, peaches, strawberries, cherries, blueberries, tomatoes, and watermelon.

Vegetables

Bok choy, cauliflower, Brussels sprouts, pumpkin, romaine lettuce, mushrooms, and yellow onions.

Unrefined Whole Grains

Rolled oatmeal, barley, and brown rice

Fatty Fish

Trout, albacore tuna.

Herbs and Spices

All-spice, basil, bay leaf, black pepper, caraway seeds, cardamom, cayenne, cloves, coriander, cumin, dill, fennel, lemongrass, mint, nutmeg, oregano, paprika, rosemary, sage, tarragon, and thyme.

Natural Teas

Dandelion, cherry, ginger, masala chai, oolong, pineapple, rooibos, rosehips, and turmeric,

Sweets and Sweeteners

Sweetener with low glycemic indexes like stevia and allulose, erythritol

Others

Baking powder, peanut butter

Chapter 3: Preparing to Practice the Anti Inflammatory Diet

Most people fail at dieting not because it is hard to do but because they did not mentally prepare or set goals when they began the regimen. By taking the time to set your goals and plan the way forward, you pave the way to keep focused and motivated when the going gets tough, which it eventually will. You create a sense of purpose and have a vision of what you would like to achieve. Is it simply enough to live a healthy lifestyle and prevent common illness and disease? Perhaps you would like to lose weight in combination with decreasing inflammation triggers in your diet? Maybe it is because you want to decrease your chances of developing heart disease?

No matter what you would like to achieve, setting a goal that is smart, measurable, realistic, and irrelevant sets you up for success. Sticking to a diet of any kind involves developing good habits to replace your bad habits. For example, instead of reaching for French fries as a snack, fill up on fruits and vegetables. The longer you practice this, the more likely you are to do it like it's second nature in the future. After a while, you will not even think about the benefits or need to keep yourself motivated to reach for the healthier alternative. It will simply become muscle memory.

Hold yourself accountable and monitor your progress. Journaling is a great way to do this as it shows you how far you have come. Every small step contributes toward your greater success. Sometimes the small steps are unclear in your mind at first, however, when you create a system where you can see their contribution and track them, you can realize their relevance.

Lose 20 lb in one week! Many of us have heard many an advertisement promoting achievements that seemed impossible if done in a healthy way. While it is certainly possible to lose 20 lb in one week, it is most often involves starving the body and creating unhealthy conditions internally. Undertaking such an endeavor creates more harm than good. Do not get caught up in the hype. Set goals that are realistic and do not put unnecessary or harmful demands on your body. This will help keep you motivated and avoid false starts.

Also plan for setbacks. No matter what area of your life that you set goals for, there will be roadblocks and hurdles to face. Do not feel dejected or let this hinder your progress in any way. Consider the possible setbacks and have a plan to get you back on track as quickly as possible should they occur. In addition to setting your goals, allow time to reassess and adjust your goals if it is needed.

I am saying this not to overwhelm you, but to impress upon you the importance of developing the right mindset to not only eat healthier, but to completely overhaul your life for a physical, mental, and emotional transformation. It is not enough to change your diet, even as important as that aspect is. To get the most out of anti inflammation diet, you need to change your lifestyle.

It might seem hard at first, especially if you suffer from

sugar addiction which we will cover a little later on in this chapter, but I guarantee you that the benefits will be worth it in the end.

Sugar and Its Effects on Inflammation

Sugar is a known trigger for chronic information as it promotes the secretion of inflammatory indicators such as CRP and the production of LDL cholesterol, which is known as the bad cholesterol.

In addition to its negative contribution to chronic inflammation, sugar can lead to weight gain, digestive issues, heart disease, type 2 diabetes, liver disease and even some types of cancers.

With so many negative effects, it is obvious that sugar intake needs to be limited and quite possibly eliminated from the diet to ensure good health and longevity. However, removing sugar from their diet can be very difficult for most of the global population.

How to Deal with Sugar Withdrawal

Sugar is eight times as addictive as cocaine. Is it any wonder that most people cannot just stop consuming it even though they know how damaging it is to their health when consumed in unhealthy amounts? You may not even realize that you have a sugar dependency because you do not consume a lot of foods that are considered high in sugar. However, there are many foods that contain hidden sugars. Examples of this include granola bars, yogurt, crackers, pasta sauce, salad dressings, breakfast cereals, and instant oatmeal.

Excessive sugar intake has been linked to obesity, heart disease, cancer, type 2 diabetes, poor dental health, and more. The reason sugar is so addictive is that it creates a cycle of chronic craving because it gives a rush of energy when consumed. That rush is quickly followed by a sudden drop in energy. Your body craves that high again and therefore, craves sugar. This creates an endless cycle if you do not put a stop to it.

Let's take a closer look at how this addictive cycle works:

1. You consume a sugary food.
2. Insulin levels become elevated and your liver converts sugar into fat.
3. When this sugar enters your bloodstream, your blood pressure rises.
4. The levels of dopamine, a feel-good hormone, increases and makes you feel happy, working similarly to how heroin does.
5. Due to the high levels of insulin, sugar levels fall rapidly, hence, creating a feeling of fatigue. This sends signals to your brain making it crave for more sugar.
6. Therefore, you consume more sugary foods.

Excessive sugar intake is not only a trigger for inflammation, it also:

- Causes bad breath and dental cavities as it promotes the development of bacteria in the mouth.
- Causes skin to age faster since it attaches itself to collagen proteins to create AGEs also known as advanced glycation end products, which

causes skin to lose its elasticity hereby creating wrinkles
- Increases the risk of developing type 2 diabetes and heart disease as it causes the pancreas to work overtime to pump out insulin which breaks down the organ.
- Increases the risk of kidney damage as the kidneys need to filter blood sugar levels.
- Make blood vessels to grow faster than normal and get tense, which creates a narrow space for blood to travel. This increases the stress on the heart and therefore elevates the risk of developing heart disease.

Sugar is a simple carbohydrate molecule, however, its effects on our bodies are rather significant. As sugar is a carbohydrate, in addition to the unhealthy dependency it creates, it is a substance that is not allowed in the anti inflammatory diet. If you are like most of the world population, you too might suffer from a sugar dependency and as such you should expect to feel the symptoms that come with the withdrawal from it. Remember that this is more addicting that cocaine.

Sugar withdrawal symptoms include:

- Headaches
- Decreased energy
- Lowered mental acuteness
- Gastrointestinal distress

The important thing to remember is that this is a temporary phase. In a few days, you will get relief as long as you stick with the diet.

Most people think that we need sugar in our diets but

fundamentally we do not. Sugar is an energy source. We can replace it with better alternatives that treat our bodies better. Proteins and fats are more powerful sources of energy. While they may not be as quick to breakdown and produce that rush of energy, their effect is more sustainable and healthier for the gut. Protein and fat can be obtained from fatty fish, fruits, vegetables, seeds, and nuts.

The anti inflammatory diet helps detox sugar from your lifestyle. You do this by removing substances from your cabinets and repairing your eating habits. While it may at first be difficult to keep away from the sugary temptation, think of the benefits in addition to the obvious of fight against chronic inflammation. They include:

- Weight loss
- Reduced bloating
- More regulated moods
- Better dental health
- Sustained energy through the day
- Clearer skin.

Helpful Lifestyle Tips on Managing Chronic Inflammation

Remember that to fight chronic inflammation, it is not enough to just change your diet. You also need to make changes in your life that will not only fight inflammation, but will also help you fight other diseases, enjoy general good health and wellness, and make you a happier, more fulfilled individual. Some solutions for living a healthy lifestyle that fights chronic inflammation are included below:

Count Calories For Better Health

Counting calories has traditionally been a way to help people lose weight. By extension, it is also beneficial in preventing the trigger of chronic inflammation. While this is a widely used term, most people only have a vague notion of what it is. Let's take a look at what a calorie actually is before we move further.

A calorie is a measure of energy, specifically the amount of energy in foods. We use it for biological functions in our bodies such as breathing, thinking, walking, and talking. Calories are not bad things as they have been portrayed to be. The issue arises when there is an excessive intake of calories than our personalized recommended intake. The body stores excess calories in the form of fat, leading to weight gain over time. The body views fat deposits as an intrusion, leading to the immune system attacking itself which causes chronic inflammation.

By counting calories, you become more aware of what you are putting into your body and thus increases your chances of managing your weight in an effective and sustainable way. The number of calories you should consume daily depends on factors such as activity level, gender, metabolic health, age, and weight. However, on average, a woman needs 2000 calories a day while a man needs 2500 calories per day.

Most times, the only thing you need to do to control your calorie intake is to lower your portion sizes. However, there are certain foods that provide the body with a lot more calories compared to others.

For the best results when counting calories are a few tips:

- Measure your calorie intake with a mobile app or online, which will help you measure your

calorie intake for the food you consume.
- Get rid of the junk food in your cupboards as most of them have high calorie counts. Replace them with healthy alternatives such as fruits, nuts, seeds, and vegetables.
- Read the labels on the food you purchase as most of them contain useful nutritional information including the calorie count per serving.
- Consume enough calories to fuel your workout or exercise regiment as dieting and exercise go hand-in-hand.
- Do not try to undercut your calorie intake as consuming too few calories will leave you feeling fatigued throughout the day.

To help you get the most out of the calories that you consume from the recipes to come in the following chapters, we have included the calorie count.

Exercising and its Anti Inflammatory Benefits

Exercising is an effective way of fighting inflammation in addition to its many benefits such as reducing the risk of developing cardiovascular disease, type 2 diabetes, and some forms of cancer. Exercise also helps lower blood pressure, improve metabolism, and control weight loss.

Several studies have shown that just 20 minutes of exercise per day helps reduce the production of pro inflammation indicators such as cytokines and CRP. Exercise also makes your body muscle release protein called IL-6 (Interleukin 6), which has many anti-inflammatory effects such as:

- Decreasing the levels of a protein called TNF

alpha, which is a pro inflammation substance.
- Inhibiting the signaling effects of a protein called interleukin 1 beta. This protein triggers inflammation.

How long you exercise is directly proportional to how much you will benefit from the anti-inflammatory properties of IL-6. The longer you exercise, the more of this substance is released. This protein's levels peak at the time that you finish your workout and rapidly decreases back to its pre-existing levels. However, the effects are long-lasting in preventing the trigger of inflammation.

How Stress Contributes Toward Chronic Inflammation and How you can Manage it

We live in a fast-paced world and avoiding stress is next to impossible. Most people feel tired, distracted, irritated, and plagued with the feeling that they are not doing enough everyday. Most people think that this is simply part of daily living and do not realize the deep impact that stress has on the development of several diseases such as cardiovascular disease, type 2 diabetes and autoimmune disorders. Extensive stress also triggers chronic inflammation.

Stress triggers a fight or flight response, which is a short-term survival response that evolution has programmed within us to keep us safe. This response triggers the release of several hormones, such as adrenaline and cortisol. Cortisol has been dubbed the stress hormone and it promotes inflammation. Therefore by remaining in a near-constant state of stress, you are essentially triggering chronic inflammation within your body.

A few ways to help manage your stress levels are by:

- Practicing meditation.

- Not multitasking. Instead, focus on one thing at a time.
- Taking a break from what you are doing if you feel overwhelmed, taking a full body analysis and identifying what is happening within it and actively bringing yourself back to a calmer, more peaceful state of mind.
- Exercising regularly.
- Getting enough sleep.
- Cultivating a healthier emotional state by practicing gratitude, compassion, and joy.
- Spending more time outdoors.
- Eating nutritious foods.

Managing your stress levels starts within yourself. Take the time to care for your mental and emotional health. Simple changes that you can make in your work and home life can drastically reduce your stress levels and therefore, your risk for several diseases including chronic inflammation.

Why Getting Enough Sleep is Important

Sleep is vital for the proper function of the body physically, emotionally, and mentally. Its many benefits include:

- Increased performance
- Elevated mood
- Improved memory

You are not at your best when your sleep has been disrupted or when you are suffering from a lack of proper sleep. Suffering from chronic inflammation likely results in disturbances in sleep pattern and receiving adequate sleep. Chronic inflammation gives rise to sleeping disorders like sleep apnea, insomnia, and restless leg syndrome.

Inflammation disrupts sleep in the following ways:

- It causes pain, which interferes with sleep.
- It causes stress when it is time to sleep. Chronic inflammation can cause an increase in the levels of cortisol which is a stress hormone, thereby increasing the chances that you will not be able to fall asleep at certain times of the night.
- It affects the sleep center of your brain. This part of your brain is called the hypothalamus. It is responsible for your sleep patterns. Chronic inflammation disrupts the signals in that part of the brain hereby disrupting your ability to fall asleep and stay asleep.
- It causes movement during sleep, which in itself, disrupts sleep. When in pain and discomfort due to chronic inflammation, the sufferer is more likely to move around during sleep time. This constant movement causes the sufferer to wake frequently hereby disrupting his or her sleep patterns.
- It affects the sufferer's ability to achieve rapid eye movement (REM) sleep, which is the part of the sleep cycle where you are in deep sleep, dreaming, and having the utmost rest. During REM sleep, endorphins, pain relief hormones, growth hormones, and healing hormones are released. Therefore, not being able to achieve REM sleep not only makes you feel less rested, but it also deprives you of these essential hormones.

The flip side of the coin is that bad sleep habits can also contribute toward inflammation. Sleep and inflammation are regulated by the same biological rhythm. We fall asleep and wake to a rhythm called the circadian rhythm. This is driven by the secretion and inhibitions of certain hormones within the 24-hour period. This same circadian rhythm regulates the immune system and thus the inflammation function. Once this rhythm is disrupted, so is the normal function of inflammation. Getting too little sleep and too much sleep trigger inflammation

To maintain a healthy circadian rhythm and thus healthy inflammation, develop and maintain a consistent sleep routine. Go to bed and wake up at the same time everyday while ensuring that you get the right number of hours of rest.

Most adults need between seven and nine hours of sleep every night. A deviation from that amount, for even one day, can trigger inflammation. Just imagine what this does to your body and immune system over a prolonged period of time. This happens because inadequate amounts of sleep cause the rise in pro inflammatory hormones. It is good to note that this effect is more prominent in women than in men.

Now that we have increased your knowledge and awareness of chronic inflammation, its causes and effects, and how we can prevent it, let's move onto those recipes that are not only great for our taste buds and good for our stomach, but also anti inflammatory. We have also included a few helpful notes on the recipes so that you can be assured that you are getting the most anti inflammatory benefits from each recipe.

If you are enjoying this book, I'd be very happy to receive a short review on Amazon. Thank you!

Chapter 4: Week 1 Recipes

Breakfast

Fluffy Banana Pancakes

Bananas are a great way to restore energy and relieve aches and pains. They contain antioxidants and a special compound called rutin that helps fight inflammation.

Nutritional Information

Calcium	246mg
Dietary Fiber	13g
Iron	6g
Potassium	1326 mg
Sodium	166m

	g
Protein	6.5g
Sugars	54g
Total Carbohydrates	85.2g
Total Fat	23.7g
Calories per serving	187

Time: 20 minutes

Serving Size: 1

Ingredients:

- 1 small firm banana
- ¼ cup of applesauce (pureed cooked apple)
- 1 tablespoon of soy flour
- ⅛ teaspoon of baking powder
- ¼ teaspoon of ground cinnamon
- ⅛ teaspoon of ground nutmeg
- 1 ½ tablespoon of olive oil
- A pinch of salt
- 5 blueberries for topping

Directions:

1. Peel and mash the banana in a bowl.
2. Add the applesauce, baking powder, flour, cinnamon, salt, and nutmeg. Mix well to form a smooth batter.
3. Heat the oil in a large frying pan over medium heat. Add three tablespoons of batter into the frying pan to make 1 pancake. Add as many

pancakes as the pan allows.
4. Cook this until small bubbles form on the top of the pancake then flip to cook the other side.
5. The pancakes should be golden brown on each side. Move the pancake from the heat and cook the next batch. Makes four pancakes.
6. Top with the blueberries to serve.

Pineapple Kale Smoothie

This smoothie is packed with proteins, vitamins, and minerals to give you energy to perform your best throughout the day. Its anti inflammatory properties suppress pro inflammatory indicators like cytokines.

Nutritional Information

Cholesterol	3mg
Dietary Fiber	4g
Sodium	149mg
Protein	8g
Sugars	13g
Total Carbohydrates	527g
Total Fat	9g
Calories per serving	187

Time: 5 minutes

Serving Size: 2

Ingredients:

- ¼ cup of diced pineapple pieces
- 2 cups of chopped kale with stalks removed
- 1 cup of soymilk
- 1 cup of sliced banana pieces
- 2 tablespoons of peanut butter
- 1 cup of ice cubes

Directions:

1. Blend all ingredients in a blender until smooth and creamy and serve immediately.

Energizing Chia Pounding

Chia seeds are packed with fiber, antioxidants, and protein, to give you energy for a productive day. They also contain omega-3 fatty acids to help fight inflammation.

Nutritional Information

Calcium	54 mg
Dietary Fiber	2 g
Iron	4.9 mg
Vitamin A	155 mg
Potassium	79 mg

Sodium	123 mg
Protein	13 g
Total Carbohydrates	13 g
Total Fat	16 g
Calories per serving	258

Time: 2 hours

Serving Size: 1

Ingredients:

- 2 tablespoons of chia seeds
- ¼ cup of cooked quinoa
- Dash of stevia
- A pinch of cinnamon
- ¾ cup of cashew milk
- ¼ teaspoon vanilla protein powder

Directions:

1. Combine all the ingredients in a jar and mix well.
2. Cover the jar tightly and refrigerate for two or more hours.
3. Serve with any toppings you desire such as fresh berries.

Nutty Chocolate Smoothie Bowl

This is a gluten-free, vegan recipe perfect for chocolate lovers. This recipe contains peanut butter, which is a source of healthy fats.

Nutritional Information

Calcium	138mg
Dietary Fiber	12g
Iron	2.6g
Potassium	1416 mg
Sodium	260mg
Vitamin A	150IU
Vitamin C	25.7mg
Protein	6.5g
Sugars	39g
Total Carbohydrates	79g
Total Fat	19g
Calories per serving	485

Time: 5 minutes

Serving Size: 2

Ingredients:

- 4 bananas
- 1 cup of ice cubes
- ⅔ cup of almond milk
- 4 tablespoons of peanut butter
- 4 tablespoons of dark cacao powder
- 2 tablespoons of chia seeds

For Topping

- 1 sliced banana
- 1 tablespoon of dark chocolate chips
- 1 tablespoon of peanut butter to drizzle

Directions:

1. Combine all the smoothie ingredients and blend in a blender until a smooth consistency is reached.
2. Microwave one tablespoon of peanut butter in a small bowl for 30 seconds.
3. Transfer the smoothie to two bowls and top with the topping.

Cinnamon Quinoa Breakfast

Quinoa is packed with protein, gluten-free, high in several essential nutrients like fiber, calcium, and potassium, has antioxidants, and is anti inflammatory.

Nutritional Information

Calcium	363mg
Dietary Fiber	8.2g
Iron	5g
Potassium	678mg
Sodium	185mg
Vitamin D	1mcg
Protein	13.1g
Sugars	0.1g
Total Carbohydrates	59.4g
Total Fat	8.7g
Calories per serving	359

Time: 35 minutes

Serving Size: 1

Ingredients:

- 1/2 cup of rinsed quinoa
- 1 cup of unsweetened almond milk
- 1 chai tea bag
- 1 teaspoon of cinnamon

Directions:

1. Bring the milk, quinoa, and chai tea bag to a boil in a small saucepan under medium heat. Once the mixture has started boiling, remove the tea bag.
2. Reduce the heat to low, cover the pan, and cook for 15-20 minutes
3. Remove from the heat and keep covered for 10 more minutes so that the almond milk can be absorbed.
4. Serve by sprinkling cinnamon on top.

Savory Chickpea Pancakes

Vegan and packed with fiber and protein, chickpeas improve insulin resistance and reduce inflammatory indicators.

Nutritional Information

Calcium	363mg
Calcium	203mg
Dietary Fiber	25.9g
Iron	8g

Potassium	1626 mg
Sodium	81mg
Protein	13.1g
Sugars	13.5g
Total Carbohydrates	81.7g
Total Fat	28.1g
Calories per serving	643

Time: 35 minutes

Serving Size: 1

Ingredients:

- ¼ cup of chopped green onion
- ¼ cup of finely chopped red bell pepper
- ½ cup of chickpea flour
- ¼ teaspoon of garlic powder
- ¼ teaspoon of baking powder
- ⅔ of cup water
- ½ avocado
- Salt and black pepper to taste

Directions:

1. Whisk together the chickpea flour, garlic powder, salt, pepper, and baking powder.
2. Add water and whisk until there are no lumps and to create air bubbles, which make the

pancakes fluffy. Stir in the onion and bell peppers.
3. In a large skillet that has been sprayed with nonstick spray, over medium heat, pour in the batter to make one large pancake. Cook for five minutes on each side or until each side is golden brown and the pancake does not fall apart.
4. Serve with sliced avocado on top.

Vanilla Smoothie Bowl

Vanilla contains a compound called vanillin, which is anti cancer, anti tumor, and fights inflammation by decreasing the production of proinflammatory indication such as cytokines.

Nutritional Information

Dietary Fiber	13.7g
Sodium	327mg
Protein	11.5g
Sugars	10.6g
Total Carbohydrates	42.9g
Total Fat	22.5g
Calories per serving	419

Time: 25 minutes

Serving Size: 1

Ingredients:

- 3 ripe sliced bananas
- ½ cup of ice cubes
- ½ ripe avocado
- ¼ cup of unsweetened almond milk
- 1 scoop of vanilla protein powder
- ½ teaspoon of raw spirulina powder
- Chia seeds for topping

Directions:

1. Blend all the smoothie ingredients in a blender until smooth, creamy consistency has been reached.
2. Transfer to a bowl and top with chia seeds.

Lunch Recipes

Balsamic Avocado Tomato Toast

Avocados lower the levels of proinflammatory indications and contain compounds that reduce cancer risk. Tomatoes are high in vitamin C, potassium, and lycopene — an antioxidant that is anti inflammatory.

Nutritional Information

Calcium	122mg
Dietary Fiber	13.7g
Iron	4mg
Potassium	1520 mg
Sodium	293mg
Protein	13.7g
Sugars	8.8g
Total Carbohydrates	51.2g
Total Fat	46.6g
Calories per serving	669

Time: 25 minutes

Serving Size: 1

Ingredients:

- 2 slices of multigrain bread
- 1 teaspoon of olive oil
- 6 thin slices of tomatoes
- ½ cup of mashed ripe avocado
- ½ cup of balsamic vinegar
- ¼ cup of chopped basil
- Salt and black pepper to taste

Directions:

1. Create a balsamic reduction by boiling the balsamic vinegar over medium heat and whisking constantly.
2. Reduce the heat to low and simmer for 12 minutes or until the liquid has been reduced to a thick consistency. Test the consistency with a spoon.
3. Toast each piece of bread then drizzle with olive oil.
4. Evenly coat the toast with the mashed avocado then layer the tomatoes on top.
5. Drizzle with the balsamic reduction then garnish with chopped basil, salt, and pepper.
6. Serve immediately.

Vegan BLT Wraps

Tempeh is a soy product and will be the bacon substitute

for this delicious wrap. This item is a close relative of tofu but is firmer in texture. It has a mild flavor so you can dress it up or down as you desire.

Nutritional Information

Dietary Fiber	3.7g
Sodium	722mg
Protein	23g
Sugars	4.1g
Total Carbohydrates	20.5g
Total Fat	26g
Calories per serving	382

Time: 15 minutes

Serving Size: 2

Ingredients:

- ½ package of ⅛" tempeh
- 4 washed and dried large leaves of green lettuce
- ½ teaspoon of olive oil
- 1 ½ tablespoon of soy sauce
- 1 ½ maple syrup
- ¼ teaspoon onion powder
- ⅛ teaspoon of cumin
- 4 slices of avocado
- 4 slices of tomato
- 1 tablespoon of vegan mayonnaise

- Black pepper to taste

Directions:

1. Add soy sauce, maple syrup, onion powder, cumin, and black powder in a medium bowl and whisk to make a marinade.
2. Add tempeh slices to the marinade and allow to soak for a few minutes.
3. Cut the bottom of the lettuce leaves into an inverted V shape to make the folding process easier.
4. Heat the olive oil in a large skillet over medium heat. Sear the tempeh on each side for three to four minutes. The edges will become blackened slightly.
5. To assemble the wraps, layer two lettuce leaves so that the bottom parts overlap in the center about three inches. Arrange the tempeh, tomato, avocado, and mayonnaise in the leaves.
6. To fold the wrap, tuck in the ends, and roll lengthwise. Cut this into two pieces and plate.
7. Repeat with the other two lettuce leaves.
8. Serve.

Quick Chicken Salad

This recipe contains grapes, which is an antioxidants, namely flavonoids and resveratrol, both of which have anti inflammatory properties.

Nutritional Information

Calcium	63mg

Dietary Fiber	9.1
Iron	4mg
Potassium	1248 mg
Sodium	1268 mg
Protein	38.7g
Sugars	25.9g
Total Carbohydrates	48.2g
Total Fat	50.3g
Calories per serving	772

Time: 10 minutes

Serving Size: 2

Ingredients:

- 1 ½ cup skinless chicken breast (cooked and shredded)
- 2 cups of halved red grapes
- ¼ cup of chopped red onion
- 1 diced avocado
- ½ cup of cashew nuts

For Vinaigrette

- ⅛ teaspoon salt
- ½ tablespoon balsamic vinegar

- 1 tablespoon olive oil

Directions:

1. Toss the salad ingredients in a large bowl.
2. Make the salad dressing by combining the Vinaigrette ingredients.
3. Drizzle vinaigrette over salad and toss until the salad ingredients are thoroughly coated.
4. Serve

Quinoa Veggie Bowl

Bell peppers are loaded with vitamin C and antioxidants like quercetin that fight chronic inflammation.

Nutritional Information

Calcium	19mg
Dietary Fiber	2.6g
Iron	2mg
Sodium	4mg
Potassium	235mg
Protein	4.4g
Sugars	1.4g
Total Carbohydrates	20.5g
Total Fat	10.2g

| Calories per serving | 187 |

Time: 45 minutes

Serving Size: 6 (1 ½ cup per serving)

Ingredients:

- 1 cup washed quinoa
- ½ cups of water
- 1 cup of chopped green bell pepper
- 1 cup of chopped red bell pepper
- ¼ cup of olive oil
- 2 tablespoons of apple cider vinegar
- 2 tablespoons of chopped parsley
- Salt and pepper to taste

Directions:

1. Light toast the quinoa in a medium saucepan over medium heat to remove any remaining liquid and to add a nutty flavor.
2. Add water and bring to a boil. Reduce heat and allow the quinoa to simmer for 10 minutes or until the quinoa is fluffy.
3. While the quinoa simmers, make the salad dressing by mixing the olive oil, apple cider vinegar, salt, and pepper.
4. Remove the quinoa from heat and chill in the refrigerator for a few minutes.
5. Add the peppers.
6. Pour the salad dressing over the quinoa mixture and toss with a fork.
7. Serve.

Tomato Cucumber Toast

In addition to being hydrating, anti cancerous, and alkalizing, cucumbers contain flavonoids, which are anti inflammatory antioxidants.

Nutritional Information

Protein	3g
Sugars	4g
Total Carbohydrates	24 g
Total Fat	8g
Calories per serving	177

Time: 45 minutes

Serving Size: 6 (1 ½ cup per serving)

Ingredients:

- 1 small diced tomato
- 1 diced cucumber
- 1 teaspoon of olive oil
- A pinch of dried oregano
- 2 teaspoons of vegan mayonnaise
- 2 slices of whole grain bread
- 1 teaspoon of balsamic glaze
- Salt and black pepper to taste

Directions:

1. Combine the vegetables with olive oil and oregano in a medium bowl.

2. Add the salt and pepper and toss.
3. Smear one side of the bread sliced with the mayonnaise.
4. Top with the veggie mixture and balsamic glaze.

Simple Lemon Tuna Salad

Lemons help improve digestion, enhance liver function, and fight acidity and inflammation in the stomach.

Nutritional Information

Calcium	12mg
Cholesterol	55mg
Dietary Fiber	0.8g
Iron	2mg
Potassium	735mg
Protein g	48.1g
Sugars	0.8
Total Carbohydrates	3.2g
Total Fat	30.7g
Calories per serving	484

Time: 10 minutes

Serving Size: 1

Ingredients:

- ⅓ cup of diced cucumber
- ½ cup of small avocado
- 1 teaspoon of lemon juice
- 1 can of 6 oz f tuna
- 1 tablespoon olive oil
- 2 leaves of romaine lettuce
- Salt and black pepper to taste

Directions:

1. Combine the cucumber, avocado, and lemon juice in a medium bowl.
2. Open a can of tuna, drain and dump into a small bowl. Flake with a fork and mix with the olive oil.
3. Add the tuna mixture to the avocado and cucumber mixture.
4. Place the tuna salad on top of the lettuce leaves.
5. Sprinkle with salt and pepper to taste.
6. Serve.

Paleo Veggie Delight Pizza

One ingredient in this recipe is mushroom and these contain several anti inflammatory components such as indolic compounds, vitamins and fatty acids. Mushrooms also contain antioxidants and anticancer components.

Nutritional Information

Calcium	147mg

Cholesterol	amg
Dietary Fiber	6.9g
Iron	4mg
Sodium	1322 mg
Potassium	1639 mg
Vitamin D	5mcg
Protein	26.5g
Sugars	13.4
Total Carbohydrates	26g
Total Fat	22.6g
Calories per serving	388

Time: 45 minutes

Serving Size: 4

Ingredients:

- 2 ½ cup of soy flour, plus more for dusting
- 1/2 teaspoon baking powder
- 1 teaspoon Italian seasoning
- ⅛ teaspoon of garlic powder
- ½ teaspoon of salt
- 3 teaspoons of baking soda
- 3 teaspoons of white vinegar
- 5 tablespoons of olive oil

- ½ cup of chopped red tomatoes
- ¼ cup sliced red onion
- ½ cup of sliced green bell pepper
- ¼ cup of sliced black olives
- 2 sliced cremini mushrooms

Directions:

1. Preheat your oven to 425 degrees F.
2. Prepare a baking sheet by brushing it with olive oil and dusting it with flour so that the entire surface is coated.
3. In a bowl, beginning making the dough by whisking in sieved soy flour, baking powder, Italian seasoning, garlic powder, and salt.
4. In a small bowl, mix the baking soda and white vinegar to make an egg substitute. Add this to the flour mixture along with the olive oil. Stir to form a dough. If the dough is too dry, add water a teaspoon at a time until the dough is soft and malleable.
5. Roll out the dough to a quarter of an inch thickness.
6. Transfer the dough to the baking sheet.
7. Bake for 10 minutes or until crust is golden brown.
8. Top with the remaining ingredients and bake for five minutes.
9. Slice and serve.

Dinner Recipes

Hearty Lentil Kale Soup

Lentils are high in fiber and magnesium. Magnesium helps reduce chronic inflammation.

Nutritional Information

Calcium	89mg
Dietary Fiber	12g
Iron	3mg
Sodium	170mg
Potassium	345mg
Protein	11g
Sugars	4g
Total Carbohydrates	29g
Total Fat	5g
Calories per serving	200

Time: 45 minutes

Serving Size: 6 (1 ½ cup per serving)

Ingredients:

- 2 tablespoons of olive oil

- 1 cup of chopped yellow onion
- 1 cup of diced carrot
- 2 teaspoons of peeled and minced garlic
- 1 cup of rinsed brown lentils
- 4 cups of water
- 1 ½ cup of vegetable stock
- 1 tablespoon of dried basil
- 2 large chopped tomatoes
- 1 bunch of kale
- 1 teaspoon of salt
- ⅛ teaspoon of ground black pepper

Directions:

1. Heat the oil in a large pot over medium heat. Saute the onions, carrots, and garlic for five minutes.
2. Add water and bring to a boil.
3. Add the lentils and simmer for 20 minutes.
4. Add the stock, basil and tomatoes. Cover the pot and cook for no more than 10 minutes.
5. Add remaining ingredients. Reduce to low heat, cover and simmer for three more minutes.

Baked Chicken Veggie Dinner

A protein in chicken called hydrolysates has many anti inflammatory effects. This making chicken a great addition to the anti inflammation diet as long as it is consumed in moderation that it. Squash is high in fiber and has been scientifically proven to lower the levels of inflammation indicators in the body.

Nutritional Information

Calcium	89mg
Dietary Fiber	8g
Iron	3mg
Sodium	680mg
Potassium	1135mg
Protein	22g
Sugars	7g
Cholesterol	80mg
Total Carbohydrates	30g
Total Fat	18g
Calories per serving	348

Time: 1 hour

Serving Size: 4

Ingredients:

- 1 pound trimmed and halved Brussels sprouts
- 1 pound diced butternut squash
- ½ cup of yellow onion
- 1 thinly sliced lemon
- Lemon juice
- 3 large minced garlic cloves
- 4 tablespoons of olive oil

- 2 tablespoons of balsamic vinegar
- 1 tablespoon of apple cider vinegar
- 1 ½ teaspoon of salt
- 1/2 teaspoon black pepper
- 1 teaspoon of ground pepper
- A pinch of freshly grated nutmeg
- 4 bone-in chicken thighs
- 1 teaspoon of fennel seeds
- 1 teaspoon of crushed red pepper
- 1 teaspoon of ground paprika
- 1 teaspoon of garlic powder
- 4 chopped fresh sage leaves

Directions:

1. Preheat your oven to 450 degrees F.
2. In a large bowl toss the Brussels sprouts, squash, onion, lemon, garlic, two tablespoons of olive oil, balsamic vinegar, one teaspoon of salt, black pepper and nutmeg. Spread the coated veggies on a large baking sheet.
3. Make the marinade for the chicken by combining the remaining oil and salt, apple cider vinegar, red pepper, fennel seeds, sage, paprika, and garlic powder. Coat the chicken in this marinade and evenly arrange the chicken on top of the veggies.
4. Bake this for 35 minutes or until the chicken and veggies are cooked all the way through. Your can check to see if it is fully cooked by inserting the sharp tip of the knife through the chicken and veggies. If clear liquid runs from the chicken, it is done. If the knife goes through the veggies easily, they are done.

5. Plate the chicken and veggies and squeeze lemon juice on top to serve.

Baked Cod and Chickpea Salad

This is a Mediterranean recipe. Cod contains an anti inflammatory agent called carotenoid, which gives the fish its pink color.

Nutritional Information

Dietary Fiber	8g
Sodium	445mg
Protein	35g
Sugars	7g
Cholesterol	69mg
Total Carbohydrates	33g
Total Fat	10g
Calories per serving	363

Time: 45 minutes

Serving Size: 4

Ingredients:

- 4 5-ounce skinless, boneless cod fillets
- 2 cups of spinach
- 1 teaspoon of olive oil

- ½ cup of pitted and minced olives
- 2 minced cloves of garlic
- 2 tablespoons of lemon juice
- ½ teaspoon of lemon zest
- ⅛ teaspoon of salt
- ¼ teaspoon of ground black pepper
- 2 red bell pepper

For the Chickpea Salad

- 2 cups of cooked chickpeas
- 2 teaspoons of olive oil
- ½ cup of chopped red onion
- 1 minced garlic clove
- ½ cup of minced parsley
- 10 pitted and chopped olives
- 1 tablespoon dried oregano
- ¼ cup of lemon juice
- 1 ½ teaspoon lemon zest
- ¼ cup of ground black pepper
- 1 ½ cup of chopped tomatoes

Directions:

1. Preheat your oven to 350 degrees F.
2. Combine the minced olives, salt and pepper, lemon juice, and garlic in a small bowl. Set aside.
3. Trim, half and de-seed the bell peppers. Arrange the peppers on a prepared baking sheet skin side down. Brush the tops with a quarter teaspoon of olive oil. Top with the spinach and cod.
4. Add the remaining olive oil to the olive mixture and spread evenly over the cod.

5. Bake this for 23 minutes.
6. To make the chickpea salad, heat the olive oil in a medium skillet over medium heat. Saute the onion and garlic for one minute.
7. Add the chickpeas, a quarter cup parsley, lemon juice, oregano and one tablespoon of water. Cook for five minutes and stir often.
8. Add the olives and tomatoes. Cook and stir until all the liquid evaporates. This should be less than ten minutes.
9. Stir in the remaining parsley, lemon zest, and black pepper. Remove the salad from the heat.
10. Plate the cod mixture and serve with chickpea salad.

Rosemary Salmon Dinner

This recipes feature yellow mustard, which is a blend of mustard seeds, turmeric, salt, white vinegar and spices. As a result of it compounds, namely turmeric, it has powerful anti inflammatory properties

Nutritional Information

Calcium	56mg
Cholesterol	50mg
Dietary Fiber	0.4g
Iron	1mg
Sodium	66mg
Potassium	475mg

Protein	22.3g
Sugars	1.6g
Cholesterol	50mg
Total Carbohydrates	2.3g
Total Fat	7.2g
Calories per serving	159

Time: 40 minutes

Serving Size: 4

Ingredients:

- 4 4-oz salmon fillets
- 1 tablespoon yellow mustard
- 2 minced cloves garlic
- 1 tablespoon chopped green onions
- 2 teaspoon of chopped thyme leaves, plus more branches for garnish
- 2 teaspoons of chopped rosemary
- ½ teaspoon of lemon juice
- Lemon slices for garnish
- Salt and black pepper to taste

Directions:

1. Prepare your broiler.
2. Prepare a baking sheet with parchment paper.
3. To make seasoning mixture, combine all the ingredients except for the salmon and garnish ingredients.
4. Place the salmon fillets on a baking sheet and

spread the seasoning mixture over the fish.
5. Broil for seven minutes.
6. Plate and serve by garnishing with the lemon slices and thyme.

Creamy Tomato Soup

Black pepper, an ingredient in this recipe, fights inflammation with the active compound called piperine.

Nutritional Information

Calcium	35mg
Dietary Fiber	1.2g
Iron	3mg
Sodium	526mg
Potassium	527mg
Protein	44.9g
Sugars	1.9g
Cholesterol	135mg
Total Carbohydrates	3.1g
Total Fat	12.2g
Calories per serving	424

Time: 30 minutes

Serving Size: 6

Ingredients:

- 4 roasted mashed tomatoes
- 1 cup of water
- 1/4 teaspoon of black pepper
- 1 teaspoon of salt
- 1/3 cup fresh basil
- 2 tablespoons olive oil
- 2 pounds boneless skinless chicken thighs, cute into 1-inch chunks
- 1 cup of coconut milk

Directions:

1. In a cast-iron pan, add the tomato, water, salt, pepper, basil, and olive oil. Bring to a boil over medium heat, stirring occasionally.
2. Add the chicken and cook for 25 minutes.
3. Remove from the heat and blend the soup in the immersion blend.
4. Add the mixture back to the pan once a smooth consistency has been reached.
5. Add the coconut milk and stir to thoroughly combine.
6. Cook on low heat for five more minutes.
7. Serve warm.

Brown Rice Bowl with Roasted Red Pepper Sauce

Brown rice is an unrefined grain item that helps fight inflammation and is high in fiber.

Nutritional Information

Calcium	75mg
Cholesterol	1mg
Dietary Fiber	4.2g
Iron	3mg
Sodium	80mg
Potassium	404mg
Protein	6.8g
Sugars	1.6g
Cholesterol	1mg
Total Carbohydrates	23g
Total Fat	8.5g
Calories per serving	187

Time: 30 minutes

Serving Size: 1

Ingredients:

- 1 cup of cooked brown rice

- ½ cup of spinach
- ½ cup of diced cucumber
- ¼ cup of cooked white beans
- 4 pitted olives
- ¼ cup of thinly sliced red onion
- 1 tablespoon of thinly chopped parsley
- 1 teaspoon of olive oil,
- ½ teaspoon of lemon juice
- Salt and black pepper to taste

For Roasted Red Pepper Sauce

- 1 roasted red bell pepper
- 1 minced clove garlic
- 1/2 teaspoon salt
- ½ tablespoon juice lemon
- 1/2 cup olive oil
- 1/2 cup almonds

Directions:

1. To make the roasted red pepper sauce, pulse all the ingredients in a blender or food processor to a thick consistency.
2. Build your brown rice bowl, but layer all ingredients on top of the brown rice.
3. Pour roasted red pepper sauce on top and serve.

Cauliflower Roast

Cauliflower helps the body get rid of waste because it contains sulphur. It also contains the compound 3-carbinol, which helps inflammation.

Nutritional Information

Calcium	68mg
Dietary Fiber	6.7g
Iron	2mg
Sodium	74mg
Potassium	884mg
Protein	5.4g
Sugars	7.3g
Total Carbohydrates	16g
Total Fat	5.1g
Calories per serving	115

Time: 1 hour, 20 minutes

Serving Size: 4

Ingredients:

- 2 pounds of cauliflower
- 1 1/2 cup of cherry tomatoes
- 4 minced cloves garlic
- 4 teaspoon of olive oil
- 1/4 teaspoon of crushed red pepper flakes
- 1/8 teaspoon of paprika
- 1/4 cup of chopped parsley
- Salt and black pepper to taste

Directions:

1. Preheat your oven to 400 degrees F.
2. Toss the tomatoes with three tablespoons of olive oil, salt, black pepper, garlic, and red pepper flakes.
3. Place this mixture in a baking tray.
4. Trim the large green leaves and stems from the cauliflower. Sit the cauliflower flat in the center of the tomatoes. Drizzle it with the remaining olive oil and sprinkle with salt and pepper.
5. Roast for an hour. The cauliflower is done when it is easily pierced with a sharp knife.
6. Remove the tray from the oven and sprinkle with parsley.
7. Cut the cauliflower into wedges and serve with a side of tomatoes.

Chapter 5: Week 2 Recipes

Breakfast Recipes

Coconut Strawberry Smoothie

Get a boost of fiber and protein with this recipe. This is especially great to power you through a morning workout.

Nutritional Information

Dietary Fiber	8g
Protein	21g
Sugars	22g
Total Carbohydrates	31g
Total Fat	7g

Calories per serving	270

Time: 10 minutes

Serving Size: 1

Ingredients:

- 1 cup of sliced strawberries
- 1 cup of coconut milk
- 1 cup of ice cubes
- ¼ cup of vanilla protein powder
- 2 teaspoons of maple syrup
- 1 teaspoon of vanilla extract
- 1 teaspoon of ground flaxseeds

Directions:

1. Blend all ingredients in a blender until a smooth consistency is reached.
2. Serve.

Beet Berry Smoothie Bowl

Beets are great for boosting the immune system to lessen the likelihood of triggering inflammation. They also purify the blood and increase energy. And the best part, they help this smoothie taste divine.

Nutritional Information

Calcium	329mg
Cholesterol	135mg
Dietary Fiber	14.3g

Iron	4mg
Potassium	1186 mg
Vitamin D	1mcg
Protein	35.8g
Sugars	28.5g
Total Carbohydrates	58.7g
Total Fat	10.1g
Calories per serving	464

Time: 10 minutes

Serving Size: 1

Ingredients:

- 3/4 cup chopped roasted beets
- 3/4 cup raspberries
- ¼ cup ice cubes
- 1/2 cup unsweetened Almond milk
- 1 tablespoon lime juice
- 1 scoop vanilla protein powder
- 1 tablespoon flax seeds
- 1 ripe banana

Directions:

1. Blend all ingredients in a blender until a smooth consistency is reached.
2. Serve.

Coconut Almond Toast With Dark Chocolate

The almond chocolate butter give Nutella a run for its money. The nutritional value is great too. Coconuts have several benefits such as being antimicrobial, analgesic, and antipyretic in addition to being anti inflammatory.

Nutritional Information

Calcium	62mg
Dietary Fiber	3.9g
Iron	2mg
Potassium	92mg
Protein	6.4g
Sugars	5.4g
Total Carbohydrates	18g
Total Fat	3g
Calories per serving	180

Time: 50 minutes

Serving Size: 2

Ingredients:

- 2 slice of whole wheat bread
- 2 tablespoons of coconut flakes
- Roasted almonds

- A pinch of salt

For Almond Chocolate Butter

- 2 cups of unsalted roasted almonds
- 1/4 teaspoon of vanilla extract
- 1/3 cup of dark chocolate chips
- 1 teaspoon of coconut oil
- 2 tablespoons of dark cocoa powder
- 1 teaspoon of maple syrup
- 1 teaspoon of salt

Directions:

1. To make the almond chocolate butter, start by pulsing the almonds in a food processor for about 12 minutes. Scrap the sides down when the almonds stick to it. Allow the almonds to reach a creamy consistency.
2. In a small pan over the lowest heat setting, melt the chocolate chips and coconut oil, stirring until smooth.
3. Add the melted chocolate and the rest of the ingredients to the almond butter and process against for two minutes.
4. Transfer the mixture to an airtight container and store at room temperature or in the refrigerator, using as needed.
5. To make the toast, spread the almond chocolate butter on one side of each piece of bread.
6. Top with the coconut flakes and almonds and sprinkle some salt.

Tofu Egg Breakfast Sandwich

Tofu is a soy-based product and is rich in antioxidants and omega-3 fatty acids, both of which are anti inflammatory.

Nutritional Information

Calcium	488mg
Dietary Fiber	7.3g
Iron	8mg
Potassium	1387 mg
Protein	52.2g
Sugars	9.4g
Total Carbohydrates	45.9g
Total Fat	46.3g
Calories per serving	757

Time: 45 minutes

Serving Size: 2

Ingredients:

For "Egg"

- 2 slabs of tofu
- 1/4 tsp turmeric
- olive oil

- Salt and pepper to taste

For Strawberry Jam

- 2 cups of de-stemmed and chopped strawberries
- 2 tablespoons of maple syrup
- water
- 2 tablespoons of chia seed.

Other Ingredients

- 2 multigrain buns
- ½ avocado, mashed
- 3 slices of tomato
- 4 slices of prepared tempeh (See Veggie BLT Wraps recipe)

Directions:

1. To make the strawberry jam, blend the strawberry, chia seeds, and maple syrup for one minute. Add water a tablespoon at a time until you reach your preferred consistency.
2. Pour mixture into a small saucepan and bring to a boil over medium heat. Simmer for six minutes or until the jam thickens.
3. Remove from the heat and pour into a heat resistant airtight container. Allow the jam to cool then refrigerate for up to a week, using as needed.
4. To prepare the eggy tofu, blot each slice with a paper towel to remove any excess liquid. Sprinkle the tofu with turmeric and salt and pepper on both sides.
5. Heat the olive oil in a medium skillet over medium heat and add the tofu. Cover the pan

and cook for two minutes.
6. Flip the tofu and cook until the edges start to brown and tofu is fluffy.
7. To assemble the sandwich, slice your bread in half and toast it. Spread jam on one side of each half. Add the mashed avocado to the other halves. Layer the tofu slices on the jam side. continue building the sandwich by adding tomatoes and tempeh slices.Close the sandwich with the other half and serve.

Vegan French Toast

This recipe contains nutritional yeast, which supports a healthy immune system and helps reduce inflammation caused by bacterial infection.

Nutritional Information

Calcium	150mg
Dietary Fiber	13.6g
Iron	7mg
Potassium	984mg
Protein	17.3g
Sugars	26.3g
Total Carbohydrates	72.9g
Total Fat	45.9g

| Calories per serving | 738 |

Time: 20 minutes

Serving Size: 1

Ingredients:

- 2 slices of whole wheat bread
- 1/2 cup of almond milk
- 1 tablespoon of maple syrup
- 2 tablespoons of whole wheat flour
- 1 tablespoon of nutritional yeast
- 1 teaspoon of cinnamon
- ¼ teaspoon of ground nutmeg
- A pinch of salt
- Coconut oil

Toppings

- Maple syrup
- Strawberry slices

Directions:

1. Whisk together all the ingredients except for the bread and coconut oil.
2. Place the bread in a shallow bowl and pour the wet mixture over it. Ensure that the bread slices soak up the wet mixture.
3. Heat the coconut oil in a large skillet over medium heat. Add the bread slices and cook both sides until they are golden brown.
4. Serve warm with the toppings.

Homemade Blueberry Waffles

Packed with antioxidants and phytoflavinoids, blackberries are high in potassium and vitamins, properties that lower the risk of heart disease, cancer, and inflammation.

Nutritional Information

Calcium	170mg
Dietary Fiber	8.5g
Iron	8mg
Potassium	755mg
Protein	16.8g
Sugars	19g
Total Carbohydrates	122.7g
Total Fat	21g
Calories per serving	811

Time: 20 minutes

Serving Size: 2

Ingredients:

- ¾ cups almond milk
- 3/4 tablespoons apple cider vinegar
- 1 tablespoon of melted coconut oil
- 2 tablespoons maple syrup

- ¼ teaspoon vanilla extract
- 2 cups of wheat flour
- 1 teaspoon of baking powder
- 2 tablespoons of flax meal (Flax seeds pulsed into a powder)
- ¼ teaspoon cinnamon
- A pinch of salt
- ½ cup of quartered blueberries
- Maple syrup for topping

Directions:

1. Preheat your waffle iron.
2. Mix the dry ingredients in a large bowl.
3. Mix the wet ingredients in another bowl.
4. Add wet ingredients to dry and mix until they are all just combined. Do not over mix.
5. Scoop the batter into your waffle iron and follow the cooking instructions of your waffle iron. Place the blueberries pieces on the top of the waffle mixture before pressing the iron.
6. Serve the waffle hot, topped with the maple syrup. These waffles can be stored in the freezer and popped into the toaster when needed.

Maple Coconut Oats

Maple syrup has a compound that has been scientifically proven to prevent inflammation. It is called quebecol.

Nutritional Information

Calcium	40mg

Dietary Fiber	23.1g
Iron	31mg
Potassium	1128 mg
Protein	12.5g
Sugars	19.4g
Total Carbohydrates	50.4g
Total Fat	98.2g
Calories per serving	1071

Time: 20 minutes

Serving Size: 2

Ingredients:

- 1/3 cup of rolled oats
- 1 teaspoon of maple syrup
- 1 cup of coconut milk

Toppings

- Coconut flakes
- 1 tablespoon of crushed walnuts
- ¼ cup of blackberries

Directions:

1. Add the oats, maple syrup, and coconut milk to a small saucepan over medium heat.
2. Reduce the heat and cook the oats until the mixture as thickened, stirring constantly.

3. Pour the oats into a bowl and serve warm with toppings.

Lunch Recipes

Curry Apple Tuna Salad

Apples are high in antioxidants that help fight inflammation.

Nutritional Information

Calcium	13mg
Dietary Fiber	1g
Iron	1mg
Potassium	436mg
Protein	30.3g
Sugars	2.9g
Total Carbohydrates	5.1g
Total Fat	11.9g
Calories per serving	255

Time: 20 minutes

Serving Size: 4

Ingredients:

- 1 pound of tuna
- ½ cup of diced green apples
- ¼ cup of chopped parsley
- 1/3 cups of vegan mayo
- 1 teaspoon of curry powder
- 1 teaspoon of salt
- ½ teaspoon of lime juice

Directions:

1. To keep the apple slices from turning brown, combine the lime juice with 1 cup of water and place the piece in the water.
2. When it is time to assemble your salad, drain the apple pieces. Add all the ingredients to a medium bowl. Mix well.
3. Serve and chill any remainder.

Broccoli Tempeh Salad

Broccoli is rich in antioxidant that deduce the levels of proinflammatory indicators like cytokines.

Nutritional Information

Calcium	176mg
Dietary Fiber	4.8g
Iron	3mg

Potassium	854mg
Protein	23g
Sugars	4.3g
Total Carbohydrates	24.2g
Total Fat	24.6g
Calories per serving	386

Time: 25 minutes

Serving Size: 4

Ingredients:

- 4 cooked and diced tempeh slices (See the Vegan BLT Wrap recipe for directions)
- 3 heads broccoli
- 2 carrots
- 1/2 red onion
- 1/2 cup of dried cranberries
- 1/2 cup of sliced almonds
- A pinch of salt

For Salad Dressing

- 1/2 cup of vegan mayonnaise
- 3 tablespoons of apple cider vinegar
- Salt and black pepper to taste

Directions:

1. Prepare the vegetables by cutting the broccoli

into bite-size pieces, shredding the carrots and thinly slicing the red onion.
2. Bring four cups of water to a boil. Add a pinch of salt and add the broccoli pieces. Cook for a minute and a half.
3. Prepare an ice bath by adding ice cubes to a bowl of water.
4. Use a slotted spoon to place the cooked broccoli pieces into the ice bath. When the pieces have become cooled, use a colander to drain.
5. In a large bowl, add the rest of the salad ingredients.
6. To make the salad dressing, whisk together all the ingredients.
7. Pour the dressing over the broccoli mistires and gentle fold to incorporate all the ingredients.
8. Plate and serve.

Loaded Veggie Sandwich

Bean sprouts, an ingredient in this recipe, contain antioxidants that lower CRP levels.

Nutritional Information

Calcium	53mg
Dietary Fiber	2.3g
Iron	1mg
Potassium	299mg
Protein	3.7g

Sugars	5.3g
Total Carbohydrates	16.9g
Total Fat	3.4g
Calories per serving	106

Time: 25 minutes

Serving Size: 4

Ingredients:

- 2 slices whole wheat bread
- 3 tablespoons vegan mayonnaise
- 1 teaspoon of yellow mustard
- 1 lettuce leaf
- 1/4 cup bean sprouts
- 2 slices of tomato
- 2 slices of cucumber
- Thin slices of red onion

Directions:

1. Toast the bread.
2. Spread mayonnaise on one side of one slice and mustard on one side of the other slice of bread,
3. Layer on the vegetables on the mayonnaise side of that slice of bread.
4. Place the other slice of bread mustard-side down on this.
5. Slice diagonally and serve.

Veggie Burger with Jalapeno Mayo

Sweet, spicy, tangy, and good for you, this veggie burger is hearty enough to fuel the rest of your day and flavorful enough to have your tastebuds singing. It is packed with anti inflammation ingredients that are easy on your gut.

Nutritional Information

Calcium	235mg
Dietary Fiber	14.4g
Iron	7mg
Sodium	447mg
Potassium	1472 mg
Protein	25.3g
Sugars	9.8g
Total Carbohydrates	87.6g
Total Fat	22.2g
Calories per serving	628

Time: 45 minutes

Serving Size: 6

Ingredients:

For Patty

- 1 cup of cooked brown rice
- 1 cup of raw walnuts
- 1/2 tablespoon olive oil plus extra
- ¾ cups of finely chopped white onion
- 1 tablespoon of chili powder,
- 1 tablespoon of cumin powder
- 1 tablespoon of paprika
- 1/2 tsp each salt
- ½ teaspoon of black pepper
- 1 1/2 cups cooked black beans
- 1/3 cup panko bread crumbs
- 3 tablespoons vegan BBQ sauce

Jalapeno Mayo

- 6 tablespoons of vegan mayonnaise
- 4 teaspoon dried jalapeno
- 3 tablespoon of lime juice
- Salt and black pepper to taste

Sauteed Kale

- 6 cups kale, torn
- 5 teaspoons of olive oil
- dash fine pepper
- 8 teaspoons of pumpkin seeds
- 3 shallots, thinly sliced
- Salt and black pepper to taste

Other Ingredients

- 6 large whole wheat burger buns
- avocado slices

Directions:

1. To make the patties, heat a skillet over medium heat and toast the raw walnuts for about five minutes or until they are golden brown. Spoon the walnuts out of the pan and into a bowl and allow to cool.
2. In the same pan over medium heat, add the olive oil and saute onions until they are translucent. Season with the salt and black pepper. Spoon out of the pan and set aside.
3. Using a blender or food processor, pulse the cooled walnuts with the chili powder, cumin, paprika, light salt, and pepper to taste. Pulse until a fine, grainy texture has been achieved. Set this aside.
4. Mash the dried, cooked black beans with a fork in a large bowl.
5. Add the cooked brown rice, walnut mixture, sauteed onion, bread crumbs, and vegan BBQ sauce. Mix this thoroughly to form a moldable dough. If the mixture is too dry, add more BBQ sauce. If it is too wet, add more breadcrumbs.
6. Divide the dough into six large patties. Press these between your palms to achieve a thickness of ¾ of an inch. Set the prepared patties on a backing sheet or plate.
7. To cook the patties, heat a few drops of olive oil in a large skillet over medium heat. Add as many pantties as can fit in the skillet when hot.
8. Cook for four minutes on each side or until the patties have become well browned.
9. Remove from heat and set aside until time to assemble burgers.
10. While the burgers are cooking make the

sauteed kale by heating olive oil in a pan and then adding all the other ingredients to a warm pan. Cover the pot and allow the kale to cook for about one minute. The kale will wilt and become infused with the flavor of the other ingredients. Turn off the heat when down.
11.   To make the jalapeno mayo, simply mix all the ingredients in a bowl.
12.   Start to assemble the burgers by halving the burger buns and toasting lightly.
13.   On one side, spread the jalapeno mayo. Top this with a veggie burger patty then some of the sauteed kale. Spread jalapeno mayo on the other bun and close the burger and serve warm.

Crunchy Quinoa Salad with Peanut Sauce

Sweet, spicy, tangy, and good for you, this veggie burger is hearty enough to fuel the rest of your day and flavorful enough to have your taste buds singing. It is packed with anti inflammation ingredients that are easy on your gut.

Nutritional Information

Calcium	93mg
Dietary Fiber	5g
Iron	3mg
Sodium	734mg
Potassium	635mg
Protein	11.2g

Sugars	6.5g
Total Carbohydrates	36.3g
Total Fat	12.2g
Calories per serving	287

Time: 40 minutes

Serving Size: 4

Ingredients:

For Peanut Sauce

- ¼ cup of smooth peanut butter
- 3 tablespoons of soy sauce
- 1 tablespoon of maple syrup
- 1 tablespoon of white vinegar
- 1 teaspoon of olive oil
- 1 teaspoon of grated ginger
- 1 teaspoon of lime juice

For Quinoa Salad

- ¾ cup of washed quinoa
- 1 ½ cups of water
- 2 cups of torn kale
- 1 cup of grated carrot
- ½ cup of chopped cilantro
- ¼ cup of thinly sliced green onion
- ¼ cup of chopped roasted salted peanuts for topping

Directions:

1. Add the washed quinoa to a saucepan and add the oil. Toast the quinoa for a minute and a half over medium heat. The water should completely evaporate.
2. Add water to the lightly toasted quinoa and bring this to a boil.
3. Cook for 15 minutes then turn down the heat to the lowest setting and cover the pot with a lip to make the quinoa fluffy in texture.
4. Remove the quinoa from the heat and let cool. Keep the pot covered for five more minutes. Remove the lid and fluff the quinoa with a fork then set aside to cool further.
5. To make the peanut sauce, microwave peanut butter and soy sauce for 30 seconds that mix for a smooth consistency.
6. Add the remaining ingredients and whisk until smooth. Set aside.
7. In a large bowl, combine the cooled quinoa with the veggies. Toss to combine then add the peanut sauce. Divide the salad and serve.

Mushroom Tofu Sloppy Joes

This recipe makes use of apple cider vinegar, which is a pain reliever for the pain of rheumatoid arthritis. It also reduces the swelling among is anti inflammatory healing properties.

Nutritional Information

Calcium	399mg
Dietary Fiber	7.7g
Iron	5mg

Sodium	501mg
Potassium	775mg
Vitamin D	63mcg
Protein	23.2g
Sugars	6.6g
Total Carbohydrates	26g
Total Fat	24.9g
Calories per serving	391

Time: 40 minutes

Serving Size: 4

Ingredients:

- 4 whole wheat hamburger buns
- 1 cup of grated crimini mushrooms
- 8 ounces firm tofu, drained and crumbled
- 2 tablespoons olive oil
- 1 cup of chopped yellow onion
- 2 tablespoon of sliced garlic
- 2 tablespoons of chili powder
- 1 teaspoon of paprika
- 2 large roasted and pureed tomatoes
- ½ cup finely chopped walnuts
- 2 tablespoons apple cider vinegar
- 2 tablespoons tomato sauce
- 1 tablespoon soy sauce
- Salt to taste

Directions:

1. Heat the olive oil in a large skillet over medium heat and sauté the onion and garlic until the onion becomes translucent.
2. Add mushrooms, tofu, chili powder, and paprika to the skillet. Cook for five minutes, stirring occasionally.
3. Add the roasted pureed tomato purée, walnuts, apple cider vinegar, tomato sauce, and soy sauce.
4. Bring to a boil and then simmer for 15 minutes.
5. Sprinkle with salt and remove from the heat.
6. Slice the buns in half and toast them. Scoop some of the mushroom mixture on the bottom half of the buns and close with the top half.

Green Bean Tofu Salad

Green beans help reduce CRP levels.

Nutritional Information

Calcium	353mg
Dietary Fiber	3.7g
Iron	3mg
Sodium	618mg
Potassium	411mg
Protein	14.8g
Sugars	2g
Total Carbohydrates	7.6g
Total Fat	7.7g
Calories per serving	143

Time: 5 minutes

Serving Size: 4

Ingredients:

- 4 diagonally sliced celery stalks
- 2 cups trimmed and sliced green beans
- ½ braised 8-oz. block firm tofu
- ¼ cup unsalted roasted peanuts
- 2 tablespoon lime juice

- ⅛ teaspoon of salt

Directions:

1. Slice the braised tofu into thin strips.
2. Toss all ingredients together in a medium bowl then serve.

Dinner Recipes

Lemon Chicken Soup

Bay leaf, as used in this recipe, has anti-inflammatory properties that help relieve joint pains and swelling.

Nutritional Information

Calcium	168mg
Dietary Fiber	16.5mg
Iron	9mg
Sodium	231mg
Potassium	1580mg
Protein	83.5g
Sugars	2.5g

Total Carbohydrates	42.5g
Total Fat	34.5g
Calories per serving	823

Time: 45 minutes

Serving Size: 6 (1 ½ cup per serving)

Ingredients:

- 1 pound boneless skinless chicken thighs
- 2 tablespoons of olive oil
- 4 minced cloves of garlic
- 1 diced yellow pepper
- 1 cup of diced carrots
- 2 diced celery stalks
- half a teaspoon of dried thyme
- 8 cups of unsalted chicken stock
- 2 cups of cooked cannellini beans
- 1 cups of spinach
- 2 tablespoons of lemon juice
- 2 tablespoons of chopped parsley
- 2 tbsp of chopped dill
- 2 bay leaves
- Salt and pepper to taste

Directions:

1. Cut the chicken into one-inch chunks and season with salt and pepper.
2. In a large Dutch oven, heat one tablespoon of olive oil the medium heat. Sear the chicken on both sides until golden brown then set aside.

3. Add the remaining olive oil to the Dutch oven then saute the garlic, onion, celery, and carrots. Stir occasionally and cook the vegetables until tender. Stir in the thyme for about a minute.
4. And the bay leaves and chicken stock and bring the mixture to a boil.
5. Reduce the heat and stir in cannellini beans and chicken. Stir occasionally and cook this for 15 minutes or until the gravy has thickened slightly.
6. Add the spinach and cook for about two minutes.
7. Stir in remaining ingredients.
8. Remove from heat and serve immediately.

Curried Veggies Over Brown Rice

Nutritional Information

Calcium	140mg
Dietary Fiber	12.4g
Iron	7mg
Sodium	332mg
Potassium	1192mg
Protein	18.8g
Sugars	8.6g
Total Carbohydrates	166g
Total Fat	30.8g

Calories per serving	996

Time: 15 minutes

Serving Size: 4

Ingredients:

- 4 cups of cooked brown rice
- 1 tablespoon of olive oil
- 1 cup of chopped yellow onion
- 1 tablespoon of grated ginger
- 1 tablespoon of minced garlic
- 1 red bell pepper, sliced into thin 2-inch long strips
- 1 green bell pepper, sliced into thin long strips
- 3 julienned carrot
- 2 tablespoons of curry powder
- 1 ½ cup of coconut milk
- ½ cup water
- 1 ½ cups of spinach
- 1 tablespoon of soy sauce
- 2 teaspoons of lime juice
- Chopped basil for topping
- Salt to taste

Directions:

1. To make the curry, heat the olive oil in a large skillet over medium heat and sauté the onions until translucent. Add the garlic and ginger and cook for 30 seconds while stirring.
2. Add carrots and bell peppers and cook until the

peppers are tender. Sti occasionally.
3. Add the curry powder and stir. cook for two minutes.
4. Add the coconut milk, water and spinach and stir to combine. Bring to a boil over medium heat then simmer for seven minutes. Stir occasionally.
5. Remove the curry from heat and add the lime juice and salt.
6. Divide the brown rice between four bowls and top with curried vegetables. Garnish with basil and serve warm.

Garlic-Infused Seared Scallops

Scallops are rich in omega-3 fatty acids, making it a great anti inflammatory food. It is also a great source of protein.

Nutritional Information

Calcium	12mg
Dietary Fiber	0.1g
Sodium	61mg
Potassium	134mg
Protein	6.4g
Sugars	0.1g
Total Carbohydrates	1.2g
Total Fat	3.8g

Calories per serving	64

Time: 15 minutes

Serving Size: 4

Ingredients:

- 1 pound large scallops
- 1 tablespoon olive oil
- 2 tbsp. freshly chopped parsley
- Salt and black pepper to taste
- Lemon wedges

Directions:

1. Over medium heat, heat the olive oil in a large skillet. Saute the garlic.
2. Blot the scallops dry with paper towels to prevent oil splatter that can lead to injury. Season the scallops with salt and pepper.
3. Add the scallops to the heated oil mixture.
4. Cook the scallops until the bottom gets a golden crust. This will take about two minutes. Flip and cook until the same happens to the other side.
5. Serve scallops over veggies, cooked brown rice or cooked quinoa. Squeeze the lemon wedges over.

Maple Garlic Salmon

High in omega-3 fatty acids, salmon decreases CRP levels.

Nutritional Information

Calcium	84mg
Dietary Fiber	0.2g
Iron	2mg
Sodium	960mg
Potassium	733mg
Protein	34.2g
Sugars	16.9g
Total Carbohydrates	19.7g
Total Fat	21.1g
Calories per serving	394

Time: 25 minutes

Serving Size: 4

Ingredients:

- 4 6-oz. salmon fillets
- ⅓ cups of maple syrup
- ¼ cups of low-sodium soy sauce
- 2 tablespoon lemon juice
- 3 tablespoon olive oil

- 1 tablespoon minced garlic
- Lemon slices
- Salt and black pepper to taste
- Freshly chopped parsley for topping

Directions:

1. In a medium bowl, whisk together maple, soy sauce, and lemon juice.
2. In a large skillet over medium heat, heat two tablespoons oil. Add the salmon, which has been blotted with paper towels to remove the excess moisture, skin-side up. season with salt and pepper.
3. Cook the salmon for five minutes or until deeply golden.
4. Flip over and add remaining tablespoon of oil. Add garlic to skillet and cook for a minute.
5. Add the maple mixture and sliced lemons and cook until the sauce becomes reduced by about one-third. Baste the salmon with the sauce.
6. Top with parsley and serve.

Pan Fried Tuna

Tuna is another fish that is high in omega-3 fatty acids, thus its great anti inflammatory benefits.

Nutritional Information

Calcium	90mg
Dietary Fiber	8.4g
Iron	7mg
Sodium	207mg

Potassium	1550mg
Protein	125.3g
Sugars	0.5g
Total Carbohydrates	9.7g
Total Fat	38.7g
Calories per serving	894

Time: 25 minutes

Serving Size: 4

Ingredients:

- 4 6-oz. tuna fillets
- 1 cup of flax meal (grounded flax seeds)
- 1 teaspoon of garlic powder
- 1 teaspoon of onion powder
- 1 teaspoon of chili powder
- ½ teaspoon of ground cumin
- 1 tablespoon of canola oil
- Salt and black pepper to taste
- Lemon wedges, for serving
- Freshly chopped parsley for topping

Directions:

1. Combine the flax meal, garlic powder, onion powder, chili powder, and ground cumin in a large bowl.
2. Season the tuna fillets with salt and pepper. Dip them in the flax meal mixture then shake off any excess before placing each on a baking tray.

3. Heat the canola oil in a large nonstick skillet over medium heat. Add as many tuna fillets as the skillet can hold without crowding. Cook on each side for about three minutes or until golden brown. Repeat with any remaining tuna fillets.
4. Serve with lemon wedges and chopped parsley.

Kale Stuffed Sardines with Roasted Carrot Sticks

This recipe is great because of the omega-3 fatty acids in the sardines and the kale.

Nutritional Information

Calcium	337mg
Dietary Fiber	1.6g
Iron	3mg
Sodium	402mg
Potassium	616mg
Protein	19.9g
Sugars	1.6g
Total Carbohydrates	11g
Total Fat	18.2g
Calories per serving	283

Time: 25 minutes

Serving Size: 4

Ingredients:

- 2 cups shredded kale
- 1 cup boiling water
- 2 tablespoons of raisins
- 2 tablespoons of pine nuts
- 1 crushed garlic clove
- ½ teaspoon of finely grated lemon zest
- 12 cleaned sardines
- 2 tablespoons of olive oil
- 1 tablespoon freshly chopped parsley
- 2 tablespoon of panko bread crumbs
- Roasted carrot sticks, for serving (see recipe in Snacks Section)

Directions:

1. Preheat your oven to 400 degrees F.
2. Prepare a baking sheet with parchment paper.
3. Put kale in a heatproof bowl and cover with boiling water. Allow this to stand for one minute before draining the water. Refresh the kale under cold running water. Squeeze to remove excess liquid.
4. Place kale in a food processor with raisins, pine nuts, garlic, and lemon zest, and pulse to a rough texture.
5. Stuff the cavity of the sardines with the kale mixture, then place on the baking tray.
6. Sprinkle the sardines with bread crumbs then drizzle with olive oil. Bake for 15 minutes or

until golden brown.
7. Serve the baked sardines over the roasted carrot sticks and sprinkle with chopped parsley.

Maple Roasted Salmon

Nutritional Information

Calcium	
Calcium	63mg
Iron	1mg
Sodium	103mg
Potassium	663g
Protein	33g
Sugars	2g
Total Carbohydrates	2.5g
Total Fat	11.4g
Calories per serving	243

Time: 25 minutes

Serving Size: 4

Ingredients:

- 4 6-oz salmon fillets
- 2 tablespoons finely chopped fresh cilantro

- 1 tablespoon vegan mayonnaise
- 2 teaspoons maple syrup
- Salt and black pepper to taste

Directions:

1. Preheat your oven to 400 degrees F.
2. Line a baking sheet with aluminium foil. Place the salmon fillets on top.
3. In a small bowl, combine the cilantro, mayonnaise, and maple syrup. Spread this mixture on top of the salmon fillets and sprinkle with salt and pepper.
4. Bake for 11 minutes.
5. Garnish with some chopped cilantro and serve.

Chapter 6: Week 3 Recipes

Breakfast Recipes

Berry Blast Smoothie

In addition to their anti inflammatory benefits, strawberries are high in fiber and vitamins and minerals.

Nutritional Information

Calcium	352mg
Dietary Fiber	29.7g
Iron	10mg
Potassium	1554mg
Sodium	229mg
Protein	22.3g

Sugars	50.5g
Total Carbohydrates	103.8g
Total Fat	23.1g
Calories per serving	663

Time: 5 minutes

Serving Size: 1

Ingredients:

- 1 cup of chopped blueberries
- 1 cup of chopped strawberries
- 1 cup of chopped raspberries
- 1 cup of soymilk
- 1 tablespoon of peanut butter
- 1 small banana
- ½ cup of chopped kale
- 1 teaspoon of chia seeds
- 1 cup of ice cubes

Directions:

1. Blend all ingredients in a blender until smooth and creamy and serve immediately.

Spinach Salmon Delight

Spinach is a dark, leafy vegetable and carries all the major benefits of this type of veggie.

Nutritional Information

Calcium	64mg
Cholesterol	37mg
Dietary Fiber	0.8g
Iron	1mg
Potassium	5134mg
Sodium	224mg
Protein	17.9g
Sugars	0.7g
Total Carbohydrates	2.1g
Total Fat	10.3g
Calories per serving	168

Time: 25 minutes

Serving Size: 1

Ingredients:

- 1 tablespoon of soymilk
- 1 teaspoon of olive oil
- 1 cup of plain, flaked salmon
- 1 cup of spinach
- Light amount of salt and pepper to taste

Directions:

1. Heat the oil in a cast-iron skillet over medium heat. Add the salmon and salt and pepper. Cook for one minute.

2. Add the spinach and cook until mixture until the spinach wilts.

Berry Berry Quinoa Porridge

Nutritional Information

Calcium	195mg
Dietary Fiber	16.6g
Iron	5mg
Potassium	544mg
Sodium	46mg
Protein	10.5g
Sugars	13.5g
Total Carbohydrates	61.4g
Total Fat	1.2g
Calories per serving	348

Time: 35 minutes

Serving Size: 1

Ingredients:

- ⅓ cup of soymilk
- 1 teaspoon of olive oil
- ¼ cup of quinoa
- 1/8 cup of cinnamon
- ½ cup of raspberries

- ½ cup of blueberries

Directions:

1. In a fine sieve, run the quinoa under cold running water for three minutes.
2. Add the washed quinoa to a saucepan and add the oil. Toast the quinoa for 1.5 minutes over medium heat. The water should completely evaporate.
3. Add water to the lightly toasted quinoa and bring this to a boil.
4. Cook for 15 minutes, then turn down the heat to the lowest setting and cover the pot with a lip to make the quinoa fluffy in texture.
5. Drain the quinoa of any excess water and return to the heat.
6. Add the milk and cinnamon. cook for 5 minutes
7. Serve the porridge warm topped with the berries.

Peanut Butter Strawberry Banana Toast

Nutritional Information

Calcium	47mg
Dietary Fiber	6g
Iron	3mg
Potassium	511mg
Sodium	2017mg

Protein	8.8g
Sugars	14.4g
Total Carbohydrates	34.6g
Total Fat	9.4g
Calories per serving	242

Time: 5 minutes

Serving Size: 2

Ingredients:

- 2 slices of whole wheat bread
- 2 tablespoons of peanut butter
- Banana slices
- Strawberry slices

Directions:

1. Spread the peanut butter on one side of each slice of bread.
2. Top the bread slices with the rest of the banana and strawberry slices.
3. Serve.

Baked Peanut Butter Oats

Nutritional Information

Calcium	58g
Dietary Fiber	4.1g

Iron	2mg
Potassium	315mg
Sodium	107mg
Protein	6.3g
Sugars	8.1g
Total Carbohydrates	22.1g
Total Fat	8g
Calories per serving	180

Time: 45 minutes

Serving Size: 8

Ingredients:

- 1 cup of rolled oats
- 1 teaspoon ground cinnamon
- 1/4 teaspoon ground nutmeg
- 1/2 teaspoon baking powder
- 1/8 teaspoon salt
- 2 ripe bananas, mashed
- 1/3 cup of creamy peanut butter
- 1 1/3 cups soy milk
- 1 tablespoon of vanilla extract
- 1 tablespoon of chia seeds
- Banana slices for topping
- maple syrup for topping

Directions:

1. Preheat your oven to 375 degrees F.
2. Prepare an 8x8-inch baking pan by brushing it with coconut oil.
3. Mix the oats, cinnamon, nutmeg, baking powder and salt in a bowl.
4. Mix the mashed banana, peanut butter, soy milk, vanilla extract, and chia seeds in another bowl. Spoon this into the oats mixture and mix well.
5. Pour the new oats mixture into the prepared baking sheet. Bake for 35 minutes or until the top is golden brown.
6. Remove the baked oats from the oven and let cool before slicing into eight pieces.
7. Serve with toppings.

Lemon Apple Pancakes

Nutritional Information

Calcium	203mg
Dietary Fiber	1.2g
Iron	1mg
Potassium	479mg
Sodium	226mg
Protein	2.1g
Sugars	10.3g
Total Carbohydrates	15.4g

Total Fat	5.6g
Calories per serving	118

Time: 45 minutes

Serving Size: 4

Ingredients:

- 1 cup of soy milk
- ¼ cup of applesauce
- 1 tablespoon of lemon juice
- 1/2 teaspoon of lemon zest
- 1/4 tsp vanilla extract
- 3 teaspoons of baking powder
- ¼ teaspoon of salt
- 2 teaspoon of melted coconut oil
- A pinch of cinnamon
- Thin apple slices for topping
- Maple syrup for topping

Directions:

1. Mix all the dry ingredients in a bowl.
2. Mix all the milk, coconut oil, and vanilla extract in another bowl. Add this to dry ingredients.
3. Fold in the applesauce, lemon juice and lemon zest.
4. Whip the batter until it becomes fluffy.
5. Heat a large skillet that had been sprayed with nonstick sprayed.
6. Scoop the pancake batter into the pan and cook the pancake until it bubbles from the top and the edges become slightly brown. Flip the

pancake when it comes away from the pan easily without sticking. Yon can cook more than one pancake at once if the skillet can handle it.
7. Plate the pancakes and serve warm with the topping.

Quinoa Fruit Salad

Nutritional Information

Calcium	77mg
Dietary Fiber	10.2g
Iron	4mg
Potassium	704mg
Sodium	7mg
Protein	8.2g
Sugars	29.4g
Total Carbohydrates	68.6g
Total Fat	3.6g
Calories per serving	323

Time: 25 minutes

Serving Size: 4

Ingredients:

- 1 cup washed quinoa

- 1½ cup of sliced strawberries
- 1 cup raspberries
- 1 cup blueberries
- ½ cup of diced mango

Maple Lime Syrup

- ¼ cup of maple syrup
- 1 tablespoon of lime juice

Directions:

1. Lightly toast the quinoa in a medium saucepan over medium heat to remove any remaining liquid and to add a nutty flavor.
2. Add water and bring to a boil.
3. Reduce heat and allow the quinoa to simmer for 10 minutes or until the quinoa is fluffy.
4. In a large bowl, mix the prepared quinoa and fruit.
5. Make the maple lime syrup by combining the two ingredients.
6. Drizzle the syrup over the fruit salad and serve.

Lunch Recipes

Spicy Brown Rice

Nutritional Information

Dietary Fiber	13.6g
Sodium	63mg

Protein	17.9g
Sugars	16.9g
Total Carbohydrates	104.9 g
Total Fat	19.5g
Calories per serving	649

Time: 15 minutes

Serving Size: 4

Ingredients:

- 1 1/2 cups of uncooked brown rice
- 1 tablespoon olive oil
- 2 garlic cloves, crushed
- 2 tablespoons of curry powder
- 2 cups vegetable stock
- 1 cup of cooked chickpeas
- ½ cup of raisins
- 2 cups of spinach
- ¼ cup of cashews
- Salt and pepper to taste
- Roasted Red Pepper Sauce (see Brown Rice Bowl with Roasted Red Pepper Sauce recipe)

Directions:

1. Heat the oil in a large pot and saute the garlic and spinach with the curry powder over medium heat for one minute.
2. Add the rice into the pot with the stock,

chickpeas, and raisins. Stir with a fork to keep the rice from clumping.
3. Season with salt and pepper. Cover the pot and bring to a boil. Reduce to a low heat and simmer for 15 minutes or until there is no more liquid and the rice is tender.
4. Toss in cashews and serve with the roasted red Pepper sauce.

Balsamic Avocado Salad

Balsamic vinegar contains the antioxidant polyphenols, which helps boost the immune system. The antioxidant also helps to protect against heart disease, cancer and chronic inflammatory.

Nutritional Information

Dietary Fiber	6.6g
Sodium	23mg
Protein	2.8g
Sugars	15.2g
Total Carbohydrates	27.5g
Total Fat	22g
Calories per serving	311

Time: 30 minutes

Serving Size: 2

Ingredients:

- 1/2 cup balsamic vinegar
- 2 tablespoons maple syrup
- 1 tablespoon olive oil
- 6 cups chopped romaine lettuce
- 1 cup halved cherry tomatoes
- 1 halved, seeded, peeled and diced avocado
- 1/4 cup finely chopped basil leaves
- Salt and black pepper to taste

Directions:

1. Make the balsamic dressing by adding the balsamic vinegar and maple syrup to a small pan. Bring to a gentle boil over medium heat and reduce by half. This will take about six minutes. Set aside and let cool.
2. Add all the other ingredients to a large bowl. Pour the balsamic dressing on top and toss the salad.
3. Serve immediately.

Collard Green Wraps

Collard greens are associated with cancer prevention anti inflammation.

Nutritional Information

Calcium	211mg
Dietary Fiber	10g
Sodium	191mg

Protein	8.8g
Sugars	3.7g
Total Carbohydrates	18g
Total Fat	36.6g
Calories per serving	406

Time: 30 minutes

Serving Size: 4

Ingredients:

- 1 medium cucumber, peeled and sliced into matchsticks
- 2 medium carrots, peeled and sliced into matchsticks
- 2 avocados, sliced
- 1 cup of sautéed tofu
- 4 large collard green leaves, ribs removed

For Vinaigrette

- 4 tablespoons of olive oil
- 1 teaspoon of lemon juice
- ¼ teaspoon salt
- ¼ teaspoon black pepper

Directions:

1. To make the vinaigrette, whisk together all the ingredients.
2. To assemble the wrap, divide all the other ingredients in the center of the collard leaves.

tuck in the ends. fold on side over and rolled lengthwise in the other direction.
3. Pour vinaigrette into four small, shallow bowls and serve the wraps. dip the wrap into the vinaigrette.

Tangy Chickpea Salad

Nutritional Information

Calcium	124mg
Dietary Fiber	18.4g
Sodium	124mg
Iron	7mg
Potassium	982mg
Protein	19.9
Sugars	13.7g
Total Carbohydrates	66.1
Total Fat	4.6g
Calories per serving	579

Time: 10 minutes

Serving Size: 6

Ingredients:

- 3 cups of cooked chickpeas

- 2 cups chopped cucumber
- 1 chopped bell pepper
- 1/2 cup of sliced red onion
- 1/2 cup of chopped olives
- Salt and black pepper to taste

For Vinaigrette

- 1/2 cup of olive oil
- 1/4 cup white vinegar
- 1 tablespoon of lemon juice
- 1 tablespoon chopped parsley
- Salt and black pepper to taste

Directions:

1. Assemble the salad by adding all the ingredients to a large bowl and tossing it together.
2. To make the vinaigrette, combine all the ingredients and whisk.
3. Divide the salad and drizzle the vinaigrette over to serve.

Easy Tuna Sandwich

Nutritional Information

Calcium	176mg
Dietary Fiber	7.4g
Iron	4mg
Potassium	1113mg

Sodium	518mg
Protein	22.6g
Sugars	14.3g
Total Carbohydrates	47.5g
Total Fat	11g
Calories per serving	359

Time: 10 minutes

Serving Size: 4

Ingredients:

- 8 slices of whole wheat bread
- 2 tablespoon of vegan mayonnaise
- 2 (6-oz.) cans tuna packed in olive oil
- ¼ cup of finely chopped red onion
- 4 leaves of romaine lettuce
- 8 slices of tomato
- 8 slices of cucumber
- Salt and black pepper to taste

Directions:

1. Open and drain the cans of tuna. Add the fish to a large bowl and flask with a fork.
2. All the vegan mayonnaise and onions to the tuna and combine. Season with salt and pepper.
3. To build the sandwiches, layer the veggies on a slice of bread, ¼ of the tuna mixture, and close with another slice of bread.
4. Repeat with the rest of the bread and serve.

Refreshing Watermelon Salad

Watermelon contains a compound called lycopene, which inhibits several inflammatory processes. It is also an antioxidant.

Nutritional Information

Dietary Fiber	1.4g
Sodium	295g
Protein	1.7g
Sugars	13.8g
Total Carbohydrates	18.2g
Total Fat	13g
Calories per serving	184

Time: 10 minutes

Serving Size: 4

Ingredients:

- ¼ cup of olive oil
- 2 tablespoon of red wine vinegar
- ½ teaspoon of salt
- 3 cups of cubed seedless watermelon
- 1 cup of chopped cucumber
- ½ cup of thinly sliced red onion
- ½ cup of coarsely chopped mint

Directions:

1. Make the vinaigrette by whisking the olive oil, red wine vinegar, and salt in a small bowl.
2. Add the other ingredients to a large bowl. Pour vinaigrette over and toss.
3. Serve.

Tuna Lettuce Cups

Nutritional Information

Dietary Fiber	3.8g
Sodium	265g
Vitamin D	117mcg
Protein	32.9g
Sugars	2.8g
Total Carbohydrates	9.7g
Total Fat	5.9g
Calories per serving	230

Time: 20 minutes

Serving Size: 2

Ingredients:

- 1 teaspoon vegan mayonnaise
- 1 teaspoon of low-sodium soy sauce
- 2 teaspoons lemon juice
- 8 ounces cubed ahi tuna

- 2 tablespoons sliced green onions
- ¼ cup finely diced pineapple
- ¼ cup diced cucumber
- ¼ cup diced avocado
- 4 whole green lettuce leaves
- ¼ teaspoon of toasted sesame seeds

Directions:

1. Combined the vegan mayonnaise, soy sauce and half of the lemon juice in a medium bowl. Toss this with the tuna and green onion. Let this sit in the refrigerator from 10 minutes to let the flavors marry.
2. In another bowl, add pineapple, avocado, and cucumber. Toss with the rest of the lemon juice.
3. Stuff the lettuce leaves in two small bowls and top with the tuna and fruit mixtures. Sprinkle with toasted sesame seeds and serve.

Dinner Recipes

Spiced Coconut Dal

Nutritional Information

Calcium	32mg
Dietary Fiber	4.3g
Iron	2mg
Potassium	375mg

Sodium	21mg
Protein	3g
Sugars	9.9g
Total Carbohydrates	17.6g
Total Fat	28.5g
Calories per serving	315

Time: 35 minutes

Serving Size: 4

Ingredients:

- 2 tablespoons of coconut oil
- ¼ teaspoon cayenne pepper
- ¼ teaspoon cumin
- ¼ teaspoon ground turmeric
- ½ cup of chopped yellow onion
- 2 minced garlic cloves, finely chopped
- 1 tablespoon peels and chopped ginger
- 1 large unpeeled grated apple
- 1½ cups brown lentils
- 1 ½ cups of coconut milk
- 3 cups of water
- 2 tablespoon lime juice
- Salt and black pepper to taste

Directions:

1. Heat the coconut oil in a large pan over

medium heat. Add the spices and cook for one minute.
2. Add the yellow onion, ginger, and garlic, and cook until soft.
3. Add the grated apple and lentils and stir.
4. Add the coconut milk and three cups of water. Bring to a boil.
5. Reduce the heat to low and simmer for 25 minutes. stir occasional
6. Add the lime juice and salt and pepper.
7. Serve warm.

Crispy Tofu with Balsamic Maple Glaze Over Brown Rice

Nutritional Information

Calcium	137mg
Dietary Fiber	7g
Iron	4mg
Potassium	599mg
Sodium	892mg
Protein	17.4g
Sugars	10.2g
Total Carbohydrates	157.2g
Total Fat	34.4g

Calories per serving	1005

Time: 25 minutes

Serving Size: 4

Ingredients:

- 4 cups of cooked brown rice
- 8 tofu slabs
- ¼ cup low-sodium soy sauce
- 3 tablespoon maple syrup
- 3 tablespoon balsamic vinegar
- ½ teaspoon crushed red pepper flakes
- 1 teaspoon of minced ginger
- ½ cup canola oil
- toasted sesame seeds for topping

Directions:

1. Blot out the excessive liquid from the tofu slices.
2. Heat the canola oil in a large skillet over medium heat. Gentle lower the tofu sliced into the oil so that oil does not splash and cause injury. Fry, undisturbed for about four minutes or until the slices are dark brown.
3. To make the balsamic maple glaze, whisk the soy sauce, balsamic vinegar, red pepper flakes and ginger in a small bowl.
4. Remove the tofu slices and place on paper towels. Pour the oil into a container.
5. Return skillet to medium heat and add the balsamic mixture to the pan and drained tofu slices to the pan.
6. Cook this until the balsamic mixture is reduced

and thick enough to coat a spoon.
7. Plate the cooked brown rice evenly between four bowls. Spoon the tofu onto the rice and drizzle the glaze over it.
8. Top with sesame seeds and serve warm.

Garlic Broccoli Soup

Nutritional Information

Calcium	66mg
Dietary Fiber	3.1g
Iron	1mg
Potassium	344mg
Sodium	1007mg
Protein	3.1g
Sugars	4.8g
Total Carbohydrates	19.5g
Total Fat	49.4g
Calories per serving	504

Time: 45 minutes

Serving Size: 2

Ingredients:

- 2 heads of broccoli, chopped evenly

- ¼ teaspoon of minced ginger
- 7 tablespoons of olive oil
- ¼ cup of yellow onion
- 1 tablespoon of diced garlic
- 1 teaspoon of oregano
- 1/2 teaspoon of parsley
- 5 cups of low sodium vegetable broth
- Salt and pepper to taste

Directions:

1. Heat three tablespoons of olive oil in a large pot under medium Heat. add the onion and garlic and all the spices. Stir and cook until the onions become translucent.
2. Add the chopped broccoli to the pot and cook for 5 minutes.
3. Add vegetable broth. Stir. Open the pod and bring the mixture to a boil. Reduce the heat and allow the soup to simmer for 25 minutes or until the broccoli becomes soft.
4. Remove the soup from heat and allow it to cool.
5. using a hand blender, until it takes on a smooth consistency.
6. Add the remaining olive oil to this and sprinkle with salt and pepper to taste. Serve warm.

Vegan Macaroni and Cheese with Cashew Sauce

Nutritional Information

Calcium	45mg

Dietary Fiber	6.7g
Iron	5mg
Potassium	517mg
Sodium	321mg
Protein	15.5g
Sugars	5.5g
Total Carbohydrates	59.1g
Total Fat	14.9g
Calories per serving	420

Time: 45 minutes

Serving Size: 4

Ingredients:

- 4 cups of whole grain macaroni elbows
- 1 head of broccoli, cut into small florets
- 1 ½ tablespoon of olive oil
- 1 cup chopped yellow onion
- 1 grated carrot
- 1 tablespoon of minced garlic
- ½ teaspoon of garlic powder
- ½ teaspoon onion powder
- ½ teaspoon salt
- ½ of raw cashews
- 1 cup of water
- ¼ cup of nutritional yeast
- 2 teaspoons of white vinegar

Directions:

1. Heat the olive oil in a medium pan over medium heat and sauté the onion with a pinch of salt. Cook until the onion is translucent.
2. Add the grated carrots and spices to the pot. Stir constantly and cook for one minute.
3. Add the cashews and water. Bring this to a boil and simmer for six minutes.
4. Pour the cooked mixture into a blender, add the yeast and vinegar and blend to a smooth consistency.
5. Add the cooked macaroni to a large bowl and pout the cashew sauce over it. Well well and serve immediately. Leftovers can be chilled for up to four days and reheated gently to eat.

Curry Cod Dinner

Nutritional Information

Dietary Fiber	8g
Sodium	0.4g
Protein	34g
Sugars	10g
Total Carbohydrates	22g
Total Fat	6g
Calories per serving	296

Time: 45 minutes

Serving Size: 4

Ingredients:

- 4 cod fillets
- 1 tablespoon olive oil
- ½ cup chopped onion
- 2 tablespoon curry powder
- 1 teaspoon finely grated ginger
- ½ teaspoon crushed garlic
- 1 roasted pureed tomato
- 1 cup of cooked chickpeas
- ¼ teaspoon lemon zest
- 4 lemon wedges
- 2 teaspoons of white vinegar

Directions:

1. Heat the olive oil in a large skillet over medium heat and sauté the onion, curry powder, ginger, and garlic for three minutes.
2. Stir in the tomatoes, chickpeas, and some seasoning. Use a wooden spatula to crush the tomato. Cook for 10 minutes.
3. Top the simmer curry with the cod. Cover and cook for another eight minutes until the fish is cooked through.
4. Remove the skillet from the heat and sprinkle in the lemon zest.
5. Plate and serve warm with, squeezing the lemon wedges over.

Baked Salmon with Almond Parsley Dressing

Nutritional Information

Dietary Fiber	8g
Sodium	0.4g
Protein	34g
Sugars	10g
Total Carbohydrates	22g
Total Fat	6g
Calories per serving	296

Time: 20 minutes

Serving Size: 4

Ingredients:

- 4 6-oz salmon fillets
- Salt and black pepper to taste

For Almond Parsley Salad

- ½ cup of chopped toasted almonds
- 1 minced shallot
- 1 tablespoons red wine vinegar
- ¼ teaspoon of salt
- 1 cup fresh flat-leaf parsley
- 1 tablespoon of olive oil

Directions:

1. Preheat your oven to 459 degree F.
2. Prepare a baking sheet by spraying it with nonstick spray.
3. Season the salmon fillets with salt and pepper. Place on a baking tray and bake for 15 minutes.
4. To make the almond parsley salad, add the shallots, a pinch of salt and red wine vinegar to a small bowl and let sit for 25 minutes.
5. Add the rest of the ingredients. Mix and serve with baked salmon.

Cauliflower Soup

Nutritional Information

Dietary Fiber	8g

Sodium	0.4g
Protein	34g
Sugars	10g
Total Carbohydrates	22g
Total Fat	6g
Calories per serving	296

Time: 10 minutes

Serving Size: 6

Ingredients:

- 3 tablespoons olive oil
- 1 cup of thinly sliced yellow onion
- 1 head of cauliflower, broken into evenly sized florets
- 5 cups of hot water
- Salt and black pepper, to taste
- 1 tablespoon of olive oil

Directions:

1. Heat the olive oil in a large pot over low heat and saute the onion until it becomes translucent.
2. Add the cauliflower, salt and pepper, and half a cup of water. Raise the heat to medium, cover the pot and cook for 15 minutes or until the cauliflower is fork tender.
3. Add the remaining hot water and simmer for 20 minutes.

4. Take the soup off the heat and use a hand blender to puree the mixture to a smooth consistency.
5. Allow the soup to stand for 20 minutes so that it thickens.
6. Reheat and add hot water to the soup if the consistency is too thick for you.
7. Serve warm. Drizzle with olive oil.

Chapter 7: Week 4 Recipes

Breakfast Recipes

Blueberry Thyme Smoothie

Nutritional Information

Calcium	45mg
Dietary Fiber	4.2g
Iron	2mg
Potassium	440mg
Sodium	68mg
Protein	5.3g
Sugars	19.7g
Total Carbohydrates	33.7g
Total Fat	2.6g

Calories per serving	166

Time: 5 minutes

Serving Size: 2

Ingredients:

- 1 cup of blueberries
- 1 cup of soy milk
- ½ teaspoon of thyme leaves
- juice of 1 small lime
- 1 banana
- 1 cup of ice cubes

Directions:

1. Blend all ingredients in a blender until smooth and creamy, and serve immediately.

Kale and Spinach Scrambled Tofu

Nutritional Information

Calcium	546mg
Dietary Fiber	8g
Iron	10mg
Potassium	1244mg
Sodium	164mg
Protein	24.6g
Sugars	2.8g

Total Carbohydrates	23.2g
Total Fat	23.7g
Calories per serving	370

Time: 15 minutes

Serving Size: 2

Ingredients:

- 14 ounces of firm tofu, drained and patted dry
- 2 tablespoons of olive oil
- 2 tablespoons of nutritional yeast
- 2 tablespoons of turmeric
- ½ cup of chopped yellow onions
- 2 cups of chopped kale
- 2 cups of chopped spinach
- light amount of salt and pepper to taste

Directions:

1. Break up the tofu with a potato masher in a large bowl until it resembles fine curds.
2. Heat one tablespoon of the oil in a large cast-iron skillet over medium heat.
3. Saute the yellow onion, kale, and spinach. Cook until they are soft. Put this mixture in a whole and place to the side.
4. In the same cast-iron skillet, heat the remaining oil. Add the tofu and cook until the tofu has lost all liquid. This should be around five minutes.
5. Add the yeast, turmeric, and salt and pepper,

and cook until the tofu is completely yellow.
6. Add the onion mixture to this. Stir and cook for half a minute.
7. Plate and serve.

Avocado Pineapple Toast

Nutritional Information

Calcium	55mg
Dietary Fiber	10.8g
Iron	3mg
Potassium	679mg
Sodium	140mg
Protein	6.7g
Sugars	10.2g
Total Carbohydrates	32.1g
Total Fat	21.8g
Calories per serving	334

Time: 5 minutes

Serving Size: 2

Ingredients:

- 2 slices of whole wheat bread
- 1 small avocado, mashed
- 1 cup of cubed pineapple
- 1 tablespoon of flax seeds
- 1 teaspoon of chopped basil, torn
- A pinch of cayenne pepper
- Salt and pepper to taste

Directions:

1. Mix all the ingredients except the bread, flaxseeds, and basil in a small bowl.
2. Toast the bread slices.
3. Spread the avocado mixture on top of each slice of bread.
4. Sprinkle the basil and flaxseeds on top to serve.

Overnight Apple Cinnamon Oats

Nutritional Information

Calcium	94mg
Dietary Fiber	10.3g
Iron	4mg
Potassium	509mg
Sodium	68mg
Protein	10.4g
Sugars	22.3g
Total Carbohydrates	62.1g

Total Fat	5.2g
Calories per serving	318

Time: 5 minutes

Serving Size: 1

Ingredients:

- ½ cup of rolled oats
- ½ cup soy milk
- ½ cup of diced apple
- ¼ cup of lemon
- ⅛ teaspoon of cinnamon
- 1 teaspoon maple syrup

Directions:

1. Combine the oats and milk in an airtight container.
2. Toss the apple with the lemon juice to keep the apple from browning. Add this to the oats. Mix this then sprinkle with the cinnamon.
3. Chill this overnight.
4. In the morning, serve by topping with the maple syrup.

Apple Coconut Muffins

Nutritional Information

Calcium	15mg
Dietary Fiber	2.7g
Iron	2mg

Potassium	113mg
Sodium	204mg
Protein	3.9g
Sugars	5.7g
Total Carbohydrates	32.8g
Total Fat	6.6g
Calories per serving	227

Time: 45 minutes

Serving Size: 8

Ingredients:

- 2 cups whole wheat flour
- ¾ cup of applesauce
- 2 tablespoons melted coconut oil
- 2 tablespoons of maple syrup
- 2 teaspoons ground cinnamon
- 1 cup of pulsed coconut flakes
- 1 teaspoon baking soda
- A pinch of salt

Directions:

1. Preheat your oven to 325 degrees F.
2. Prepare your muffin tin by insert muffin cups.
3. Mix all the ingredients in a large bowl.
4. Fill the muffin cups to up to three-quarters full.
5. Bake for 25 minutes until the top is golden brown.

6. Remove the muffins from the oven and allow to cool then serve. These can be stored in an airtight container for a week.

Banana Pancakes with Blackberry Compote

Nutritional Information

Calcium	44mg
Dietary Fiber	6.5g
Iron	1mg
Potassium	384mg
Sodium	710mg
Protein	2.4g
Sugars	19.9g
Total Carbohydrates	36.1g
Total Fat	0.7g
Calories per serving	150

Time: 20 minutes

Serving Size: 2

Ingredients:

- 1 bananas
- ¼ cup of applesauce
- 1 ½ tablespoons whole wheat flour
- ½ teaspoon vanilla extract
- ⅛ teaspoon baking soda

- ⅛ teaspoon of cinnamon
- A pinch of salt
- 1 cup frozen blackberries
- 1 tablespoons maple syrup

Directions:

1. Peel and pure the ripe banana in a food processor.
2. Mix in the applesauce.
3. Add the flour, vanilla extract, baking soda, cinnamon, and salt to the food processor. Puree to a smooth consistency.
4. Heat up a large skillet that has been sprayed with nonstick spray over medium heat. Pour the batter into the skillet.
5. When the pancakes form bubbles on the top, flip to the other side and cook until golden brown.
6. To make the blackberry compote, place the frozen berries in a small saucepan over medium heat. Add the maple syrup when the berries begin to soften. Break up the berries with a wooden spatula and cook for one minute.
7. Plate your pancakes, top with the blackberry compote, and serve warm.

Orange Raisin Scones

Nutritional Information

Calcium	3mg
Dietary Fiber	0.6g
Potassium	36mg

Sodium	372mg
Protein	1.1g
Sugars	4.9g
Total Carbohydrates	7.1g
Total Fat	2.7g
Calories per serving	53

Time: 20 minutes

Serving Size: 8

Ingredients:

- 1 cup almond flour
- ⅛ teaspoon of salt
- ½ teaspoon baking soda
- ¼ cup raisins
- ¼ cup dark chocolate chips
- 1 teaspoon orange zest
- 1 tablespoon of applesauce

Directions:

1. Preheat your oven to 375 degrees F.
2. Prepare a baking sheet with parchment paper.
3. Combine the almond flour, salt, baking soda, raisins, chocolate chips, and orange zest in a large bowl.
4. Mix the applesauce with the dry ingredients.
5. Knead the dough with your hand for even

distribution of the ingredients.
6. Form a large circle with the dough about half an inch thick.
7. Cut the circle into eight pieces like a pizza and transfer the pieces to the baking sheet.
8. Bake for 10 minutes.

Lunch Recipes

Chickpea Salad Sandwich

Nutritional Information

Calcium	149.2mg
Dietary Fiber	14g
Vitamin A	23.2µg
Vitamin C	5.3mg
Vitamin B6	1.1mg
Vitamin B12	0µg
Vitamin D	0µg
Iron	4.5mg
Magnesium	67.8mg
Potassium	382.1mg
Protein	11.4g
Sugars	4.2g
Total Carbohydrates	54.3g
Total Fat	12.2g

Calories per serving	384

Time: 10 minutes

Serving Size: 2 (2 sandwiches)

Ingredients:

- 1 ½ cups of cooked chickpeas
- 1 tablespoon vegan mayonnaise
- 1 tablespoon lemon juice
- 4 slices of whole grain or multigrain bread
- Romaine lettuce
- Light amount of salt and black pepper to taste

Directions:

1. Mash the chickpeas in a medium bowl.
2. Combine the mashed chickpeas mayonnaise, lemon juice, salt and pepper.
3. Assemble the sandwich by adding the lettuce on once slice of bread and topping it with the chickpea mixture followed by another slice of bread.

Surprise Tuna Salad

Nutritional Information

Calcium	51mg
Dietary Fiber	14.7g
Iron	2mg
Potassium	1382mg

Protein	35.8g
Sugars	2.5g
Total Carbohydrates	20.5g
Total Fat	48.2g
Calories per serving	640

Time: 10 minutes

Serving Size: 2

Ingredients:

- 2 medium avocados
- 1 5-oz can of tuna
- 1 3.75-oz can of skinless boneless sardines in olive oil
- 1 stick of finely chopped celery
- 1/4 cup of diced red onion
- 1 teaspoon of lemon juice,
- 4 romaine lettuce leaves
- Salt and black pepper to taste

Directions:

1. Cut avocados in half. Remove the pits and skin. Place in a medium bowl and mash with a fork. Ensure that there are no lumps.
2. Open a can of tuna, drain and dump the contents into the bowl. Do the same with the sardines, except keep a very small amount of olive oil.
3. Add the rest of the ingredients except for the

romaine lettuce. Make the contents with a form and mix thoroughly.
4. Serve over romaine lettuce.

Chicken Watermelon Salad

Nutritional Information

Calcium	53mg
Dietary Fiber	2.1g
Iron	2mg
Potassium	562mg
Protein	24.1g
Sugars	17.9g
Total Carbohydrates	23.4g
Total Fat	15.9g
Calories per serving	324

Time: 15 minutes

Serving Size: 4

Ingredients:

- 2 cups skinless, boneless rotisserie chicken breast, shredded
- 4 cups cubed watermelon
- 1/3 cup thinly sliced red onion
- 2 tablespoons chopped fresh mint

- 1 cup of arugula
- 1/4 cup sliced toasted almonds
- 2 tablespoons of olive oil
- 2 tablespoons of lemon juice
- Salt and black pepper to taste

Directions:

1. Make the dressing by whisking the olive oil, lemon juice, salt and black pepper.
2. Combine all other ingredients in a large bowl and toss with the dressing.
3. Serve.

Orange Pomegranate Salad

Nutritional Information

Calcium	59mg
Dietary Fiber	6.6g
Iron	1mg
Potassium	548mg
Protein	3.2g
Sugars	14.1g
Total Carbohydrates	23.4g
Total Fat	14.4g

| Calories per serving | 218 |

Time: 10 minutes

Serving Size: 4

Ingredients:

- 2 oranges, peeled and divided into wedges
- 2 tablespoon of orange juice
- 1/2 cup pomegranate arils
- 1 cup of diced avocado
- 2 tablespoons olive oil
- 2 tablespoons chopped shallots
- 1/4 teaspoon of salt
- 1/4 teaspoon black pepper
- 2 cups of Brussels sprouts

Directions:

1. Make the dressing for this salad by whisking together the orange juice, olive oil, salt and pepper. Set aside.
2. Combine the rest of the ingredients into a large bowl and toss with the orange dressing.
3. Serve.

Veggies Sandwich with White Bean Spinach Butter

Nutritional Information

| Calcium | 392mg |
| Dietary Fiber | 22.8g |

Iron	14mg
Potassium	2116mg
Protein	39.7g
Sugars	6.7g
Total Carbohydrates	92.7g
Total Fat	17g
Calories per serving	660

Time: 10 minutes

Serving Size: 4

Ingredients:

- 8 slices of whole wheat bread
- 2 cups of cooked white beans
- 3 cups of chopped spinach
- 1 teaspoon ground cumin
- 1 teaspoon ground coriander
- 1/8 teaspoon salt
- 4 green lettuce leaves
- cucumber slices
- tomatoes slices
- ½ cup of crushed, unsalted peanuts
- Salt and black pepper to taste

Directions:

8. To make the white bean spinach butter, add the white beans, spinach, cumin, coriander, salt

and pepper together. Blend until a smooth consistency is reached.
9. To assemble the sandwich, lightly toast the bread. Spread the white bean spinach butter on one side of the bread and layer with two lettuce leaves and the rest of the ingredients.
10. Close the sandwich with another slice of bread. Repeat with the rest of the bread and serve.

Quinoa Burrito Bowl

Nutritional Information

Calcium	60mg
Dietary Fiber	9.8g
Iron	5mg
Potassium	938mg
Protein	12.7g
Sugars	2.7g
Total Carbohydrates	47.3g
Total Fat	7.3g
Calories per serving	295

Time: 10 minutes

Serving Size: 6

Ingredients:

- 1 cup of cooked quinoa
- 1 cup diced tomato
- 3 cups chopped Romaine lettuce
- 1 cup of corn
- 1 cup of black beans
- 1 cup of diced avocado
- 2 tablespoons chopped fresh cilantro leaves

For Creamy Dressing

- 1 cup vegan mayonnaise
- ½ tablespoon cayenne pepper
- ½ tablespoon of paprika
- 1 teaspoon of minced garlic, pressed
- 1 tablespoon of lime juice
- Salt and black pepper to taste.

Directions:

1. To make the creamy dressing, whisk all the ingredients together.
2. To assemble the burrito bowl, spoon quinoa to the bottom of a small bowl then layer the other ingredients on top. Drizzle with the creamy sauce and serve.

Vegan Green Mayo Sandwiches

Nutritional Information

Calcium	122mg
Dietary Fiber	5.6g
Iron	3mg

Potassium	361mg
Protein	9.2g
Sugars	6.3g
Total Carbohydrates	32.4g
Total Fat	9.7g
Calories per serving	246

Time: 10 minutes

Serving Size: 4

Ingredients:

- 8 slices of whole wheat bread
- avocado slices
- tomato slices
- cucumber slices
- red onion, thinly sliced
- 4 romaine lettuce leaves

For Green Mayonnaise

- ½ cup vegan mayonnaise
- 1/3 cup basil
- 1/3 cup tarragon
- 1/3 cup chopped green onion
- 1 tablespoon of minced cloves
- 2 anchovy fillets
- Zest and juice of 1/2 lemon
- Salt and black pepper to taste

Directions:

1. To make the geren mayonnaise, combine all the ingredients except the lemon juice in a food processor and puree until smooth. Add the lemon juice and mix in. Keep this mixture chilled until needed.
2. To assemble the sandwich, toast the bread and lay one side of all the bead with the green mayonnaise. top one slice of bread with the veggies followed by another slice of bread. Repeat until all the bread has been used.
3. Serve.

Dinner Recipes

Veggie Pumpkin Chili

This is a hearty and satisfying recipe, and is especially great on rainy days.

Nutritional Information

Calcium	211mg
Dietary Fiber	28.7g
Iron	13mg
Potassium	4354mg
Sodium	2672mg
Protein	34.7g

Sugars	20.6g
Total Carbohydrates	127.6g
Total Fat	9.3g
Calories per serving	723

Time: 1 hour, 30 minutes

Serving Size: 4

Ingredients:

- 3 cups of soaked red beans
- 3 cups of chopped yellow onions
- 1 cup of dried red bell peppers
- 2 tablespoons of olive oil
- 2 large mashed tomatoes
- 2 cups of pureed pumpkin
- 1 cup of lightly salted veggie broth
- 4 teaspoons dried oregano
- 2 teaspoons of dried thyme

Directions:

1. Saute the yellow onions and bell peppers in olive oil for five minutes in a large pot.
2. Drain the red beans and all it to the onion/pepper mixture. Break up the red beans with a wooden spatula and cook the mixture for five to seven minutes.

3. Add the other ingredients. Bring it to a boil and simmer for 50 minutes.
4. Remove the lid and simmer until cooked.
5. Serve warm.

Garlic Salmon Bake

Nutritional Information

Calcium	109mg
Dietary Fiber	2.1g
Iron	2mg
Potassium	950mg
Sodium	292mg
Protein	46.3g
Sugars	6.8g
Total Carbohydrates	24.2g
Total Fat	38.3g
Calories per serving	611

Time: 30 minutes

Serving Size: 4

Ingredients:

- 3 minced cloves of garlic

- 2 lemons, thinly sliced
- 2 pounds of salmon fillet
- Kosher salt
- 5 tablespoons of olive oil
- 2 tablespoons of maple syrup
- 1 teaspoon of chopped thyme
- 1 teaspoon of dried oregano
- Salt and black pepper to taste
- ½ teaspoon of chopped parsley, for garnish

Directions:

1. Preheat your oven to 350 degree F.
2. Prepare a baking sheet by placing foil in the center and brushing it with olive oil. Place the lemon slices in the center of the foil in an even layer.
3. Season the salmon fillets with the salt and black peppers. Place the fillets on top of the lemon slices.
4. In a small bowl, mix the remaining ingredients except for the garnish and pour this over the salmon fillets.
5. Fold the foil over the salmon and bake for 25 minutes.
6. Broil for another two minutes.
7. To serve, plate and garnish with parsley.

Apple Carrot Soup

Nutritional Information

Calcium	53mg

Dietary Fiber	5g
Iron	2mg
Potassium	334mg
Sodium	1204mg
Protein	1.5g
Sugars	14.4g
Total Carbohydrates	22g
Total Fat	7.7g
Calories per serving	150

Time: 20 minutes

Serving Size: 2

Ingredients:

- 1 deseeded and chopped apple
- 1 cup julienned carrots
- 4 cups water
- 1 tablespoon of minced garlic
- 1 teaspoon of dried oregano
- 1 teaspoon of dried basil
- ½ teaspoon of cayenne pepper
- ½ teaspoon cinnamon
- ½ teaspoon of nutmeg
- ¼ cups of coconut milk
- 1 tsp salt

Directions:

1. Bring the water to a boil in a medium saucepan over medium heat. Add the garlic and spices. Cook for five minutes.
2. Add apples, carrots, and salt. Cook for seven minutes or until apples are mushy.
3. Take this off the heat and let it cool.
4. Blend the mixture in a blender until a smooth consistency is reached. Return the mixture to the pot.
5. Reheat over medium heat and add the coconut milk. Stir to mix the ingredients.
6. Cook until the soup is warm then serve.

Curry Coconut Fish

Nutritional Information

Calcium	73mg
Dietary Fiber	4.1g
Iron	5mg
Potassium	1186mg
Sodium	207mg
Protein	39.8g
Sugars	4.9g
Total Carbohydrates	12.8g
Total Fat	33.4g

Calories per serving	496

Time: 20 minutes

Serving Size: 4

Ingredients:

- 600g of tuna fillet, cut into 1" pieces
- 2 tablespoon of chopped garlic
- 1 tablespoon of finely chopped ginger
- 2 teaspoon of olive oil
- ½ cup of chopped yellow onion
- 2 teaspoon ground turmeric
- 2 teaspoons of coriander
- 1 tsp ground cumin
- 1/4 tsp ground cloves
- 6 green cardamom pods, cracked
- 1 tablespoon of curry powder
- 2 cups of coconut milk
- 1 cup fish stock
- ½ tablespoon of lime juice
- salt to taste

Directions:

1. Heat the olive oil in a deep skillet over medium head and saute the onion, ginger and garlic until the onions become translucent.
2. Add all the other spices and cook for two minutes, stirring occasionally.
3. Add the coconut milk and fish stock and bring this to a boil. Simmer for 10 minutes.
4. Add the tuna and cook for six minutes.
5. Remove the pot from the heat and season with

lime and salt.
6. Serve over cooked quinoa, brown rice or steamed veggies.

Whole Baked Mackerel Spiced with Ginger

Nutritional Information

Calcium	83mg
Dietary Fiber	6.4g
Iron	5mg
Potassium	875mg
Sodium	88mg
Protein	24.7g
Sugars	3.9g
Total Carbohydrates	27.7g
Total Fat	51g
Calories per serving	635

Time: 50 minutes

Serving Size: 2

Ingredients:

- 4 sliced lemons
- ½ cup of thinly sliced ginger

- ½ tablespoon of minced garlic
- 1 cup coriander leaves
- 1/3 cup olive oil
- 2 whole cleaned mackerel
- Salt and pepper to taste
- Thinly sliced spring onion for topping

Directions:

1. Preheat your oven to 350 degrees F.
2. Prepare two large piece of foil and divide the lemon slice, ginger, garlic, coriander leaves, and olive oil between the two pieces.
3. Top with the two fish then add remaining lemon slices, ginger, garlic, coriander leaves, and olive oil. Season the fish with salt and pepper.
4. Seal the foil to trap the steam, place the two packages on a baking tray and bake for 30-40 minutes.
5. Remove from the oven, place each parcel on a place, open and top with spring onions.
6. Serve.

Black Bean Soup

Nutritional Information

Calcium	271mg
Dietary Fiber	30.4
Iron	11mg
Potassium	2990mg

Sodium	69mg
Protein	42.8g
Sugars	6.2g
Total Carbohydrates	128.8g
Total Fat	3g
Calories per serving	691

Time: 20 minutes

Serving Size: 4

Ingredients:

- 4 cups of cooked black beans
- ¼ cup of chopped yellow onions
- 1 cup of diced red tomatoes
- 1/2 cup chopped fresh cilantro
- 2 teaspoon of ground cumin
- 1 teaspoon of minced garlic
- 1½ teaspoons fresh lime juice
- Salt and pepper to taste

Directions:

1. Add all the ingredients together in a medium saucepan and place under medium heat. Bring to a boil the simmer over low heat for 10 minutes. Stir occasionally.
2. Serve warm.

Steamed Cod

Nutritional Information

Calcium	22mg
Dietary Fiber	1g
Iron	1mg
Potassium	116mg
Sodium	562g
Protein	21.2g
Sugars	0.8g
Total Carbohydrates	4.2g
Total Fat	1.2g
Calories per serving	118

Time: 20 minutes

Serving Size: 4

Ingredients:

- 4 6-oz skinless cod fillets
- ½ cup of water
- 3 tablespoons rice wine vinegar
- 2 tablespoons soy sauce
- 2 tablespoons finely grated ginger
- 6 chopped scallions
- Salt and black pepper to taste

Directions:

1. Combine all the ingredients except for the scallions, cod, salt, and black pepper in a large skillet.
2. Season the cod with salt and black pepper and place in the vinegar mixture. Bring this to a boil over medium heat then gently simmer over low heat. Cover the skillet and cook for seven minutes.
3. Add the scallions and cook for two more minutes.
4. Serve warm.

Chapter 8: Snack Recipes

The picture that enters most people's heads when they hear the term 'snacking' is of an overweight individual stuffing their face with copious amounts of junk food. It is about time that image is exchanged for a new and improved one because snacking does not have to be an unhealthy habit. In fact, it can help supplement your diet so that you get all the essential nutrition you need throughout the day.

Snacking, by definition is a small amount of food ingested between the regular meals of breakfast, lunch, and dinner that is easily and quickly digested by the body.

The Benefits of Snacking

- Snacking helps in weight loss management. It make be a long time in between the regular meals and hunger can arise. This leads to the

body storing fat as it goes into survival mode. Prevent this by snacking on healthy, anti inflammatory snacks.
- It increases and maintains your energy levels throughout the day by providing a source of energy
- It stabilizes your mood. Snacks that are rich in omega-3 fatty acids are especially great at fighting depression and anxiety to leave you happier throughout the day.
- It helps you control cravings. About four hours after your last meal, your blood sugar levels decrease, thus resulting in a loss of energy. This slows down your metabolism and thus contributes to cravings. As most people will reach for a sugary food as it is a quick source of energy, the negative consequence of this will be experience. Prevent this with a nutritious snack.
- Snacking prevents bloating, gas and digestive cramps.
- Snacking helps you maintain a balanced diet. Your main meals may not have been balanced. Snacking can introduced the essential vitamins, minerals, proteins, fibers, and other nutrients that you may have missed.

Tips For Effective Anti Inflammation Snacking

- Be sure to watch the salt and sugar content of the snack that you indulge in as well as the calorie content.
- Keep the portions small.
- Plan your snacks ahead of time so that you have healthy options that are anti inflammatory. Keep

these nearby so that you can reach for them easier if the need arises.
- Do not snack too frequently. Try to limit snacking to only once between main meals.
- Listen to your body and respond to your hunger signal. consider if this is a physical need or whether it is an emotion response. Emotional snack is should not be promoted and thus, you should try to avoid snacking in those instances.

Cinnamon Apple Chips

Nutritional Information

Dietary Fiber	2g
Potassium	100mg
Protein	0g
Sugars	9g
Total Carbohydrates	13g
Total Fat	0g
Calories per serving	50

Time: 2 hours, 30 minutes

Serving Size: 2 (approximately 24 chips)

Ingredients:

- Two large gala apples

- Cinnamon

Directions:

4. Preheat your oven to 225 degrees F.
5. Prepare two baking sheets with parchment paper.
6. Quarter the apples, discard the seed and slice each quarter thinly.
7. Sprinkle the slices with cinnamon lightly and toss so that each slice is coated.
8. Place the apple slices of the prepared sheets in a skin layer with the sliced evenly spaced.
9. Bake the slices for two hours, flipping them at the one hour mark.
10. Cool the chips completely before serving.

Nutty Trail Mix

Time: 45 minutes

Serving Size: 5

Ingredients:

- 1 cup of raw almonds
- 1 cup of pistachios
- ½ cup of flaxseeds
- ½ cup of raisins
- 1 teaspoon of chili powder
- ½ teaspoon of cinnamon
- 2 tablespoons of olive oil

Directions:

1. Preheat your oven to 350 degrees F.
2. Prepare a baking sheet with parchment paper.
3. Combine all ingredients in a large plastic bag and shake well until all is thoroughly mixed.
4. Dump the mixture on the prepared sheet and back for 15-20 minutes.
5. Remove the mixture from the oven, stir and place it back in the oven to bake for 10 more minutes.
6. Cool the mixture completely before serving
7. Any leftover can be stored in an airtight container.

Spicy Quinoa Crackers

This gluten-free, low-carb nutritional snack is the perfect is the perfect pairing with savory dips and has a slight nutty flavor due to the presence of all spice. The presence of black pepper gives this snack a nice kick for people who love a little fire in their food.

Nutritional Information

Dietary Fiber	4.3g
Sodium	299.3 mg
Protein	4.3g
Sugars	0g
Total Carbohydrates	22.5g
Total Fat	3.3g

Calories per serving	138

Time: 40 minutes

Serving Size: 8

Ingredients:

- 2 ¼ cup of quinoa flour plus additional for rolling
- 1 teaspoon of olive oil
- 1 teaspoon of ground black pepper
- 1 teaspoon of salt
- ¾ cup of warm water

Directions:

1. Preheat your oven to 375 degrees F.
2. Whisk together the dry ingredients and half a teaspoon of salt in a medium bowl. Create a well in the center and pour in the wet ingredients. Mix well so that all the ingredients come together in soft dough.
3. Prepare a rolling station by lightly dusting two baking mats or parchment paper and rolling pin with the additional flour. Roll half of the dough first to one-sixteenth inch thick.
4. Slice the rolled dough into one inch squares until a sharp knife or pizza cutter. Prick the center of each square with a fork.
5. Sprinkle the top with a quarter teaspoon of salt. pat the salt gently into the dough
6. Repeat with the remaining dough.
7. Place book baking mats onto a baking sheet and bake for about 20 minutes or until the crackers

are golden brown. They will have a crunchy feel.
8. Cool the crackers completing before serving. The crackers can be stored in an airtight container for more than one week.

Vegan Candied Pecans

Low in sugar, pecans help improve blood sugar levels and maintain energy levels throughout the day in addition to making your brain work better while lowering the risk of developing dementia and Alzheimewr's disease. They also contain properties that are anti inflammatory and aid in weight loss. This snack is quick and easy to make and clearly good for you.

Nutritional Information

Dietary Fiber	1.4g
Sodium	36.4mg
Protein	1.2g
Sugars	0.5g
Total Carbohydrates	2.1g
Total Fat	9.7g
Calories per serving	94

Time: 30 minutes

Serving Size: 8

Ingredients:

- 1 cup of chopped pecans
- 1 teaspoon of cinnamon
- 1.4 teaspoon of allspice
- 3 tablespoons of erythritol
- ⅛ teaspoon salt
- 1 tablespoon of water

Directions:

1. Prepare a heat-resistant flat tray. Coat with non-stick spray.
2. Mix the erythritol, salt, allspice and cinnamon in a small bowl then incorporate the water.
3. Add the pecans to a small pan and cook for about three minutes over medium heat. Stir this frequently. Add the spice mixture. Now stir constantly and ensure that all the pecan pieces are thoroughly coated.
4. Transfer the coated pecans to the prepared tray, spreading them into a flat even layer.
5. Cool completely so that the pecans harden (become candied). The pecans will become crunch in about 15 minutes buy the texture is best if you wait for a few hours
6. Break up the pecans into clumps. Serve.

4-Ingredient Kale Chips

Kale is a dark, green leafy vegetables and it is packed with the nutritional punch these types of veggies are known for. If you are a potato chip lover, here is the perfect healthy, anti inflammatory alternative. All types of kale will work for this recipe except for baby kale.

Nutritional Information

Calcium	13.3g
Dietary Fiber	1.5g
Iron	13.3g
Sodium	102.5g
Protein	2.5g
Sugars	0g
Total Carbohydrates	6g
Total Fat	1g
Calories per serving	38

Time: 30 minutes

Serving Size: 4

Ingredients:

- 1 tablespoon of olive oil
- 2 tablespoons of vinegar
- ½ teaspoon of salt
- 1 bunch of kale such as curly kale

Directions:

1. Preheat your oven to 350 degrees F.
2. Prepare a baking sheet with parchment

paper
3. Wash the kale and pat the leaves dry. Slice the stalk from the center and tear the kale leaves in even pieces of your desire. Be mindful of the fact that they will shrink during the backing process.
4. Toss the kale leaf pieces with the rest of the ingredients, leaving a small amount of salt to sprinkle on top of kale. Use your hands to ensure that the leaves are well coated. This will take a minute or two.
5. Spread kale leaves in a single layer on the baking sheet. sprinkle with the remaining salt.
6. Bake for upto 10 minutes or until the leaves are crunchy.
7. Serve immediately. The leaves can be stored in an airtight container for up to one week.

Sweet and Spicy Mango Salsa

This snack is sweet and spicy and will make your taste buds sing in addition to supplying you with many vitamins and minerals. You can serve them with whole grain chips or any other chips that comply with the anti inflammatory diet.

Nutritional Information

Calcium	23.6mg
Dietary Fiber	2.5g
Vitamin A	77.9µg
Vitamin C	51.1mg

Vitamin B6	0.2mg
Iron	0.4mg
Magnesium	14mg
Potassium	239.9mg
Protein	1.2g
Sugars	12.5g
Total Carbohydrates	16.1g
Total Fat	0.4g
Calories per serving	64

Time: 20 minutes

Serving Size: 4

Ingredients:

- 2 ripe but firm mangos, cubed
- ½ small red onion, minced
- 1 small lime, juiced
- A pinch of salt
- 2 tablespoons of chopped cilantro
- ½ jalapeno pepper, diced

Directions:

1. Combine all the ingredients in a large bowl.
2. Taste and adjust the flavors to make this as sweet, sour or as spicy as desired.
3. Let this sit for 15 minutes at room

temperature.

Berry Avocado Popsicles

Nutritional Information

Dietary Fiber	2.8g
Protein	1.8g
Total Carbohydrates	5.9g
Total Fat	13.2g
Calories per serving	152

Time: 5 hours, 30 minutes

Serving Size: 8

Ingredients:

- 2 large ripe avocados, diced
- 1 ½ cups soymilk
- 1 teaspoon erythritol
- ½ cup water
- 1 cup fresh blueberries or raspberries
- 1 teaspoon vanilla extract

Directions:

1. Blend all the ingredients in a blender until smooth. If the mixture is too thick, add more milk by the tablespoon until the desired consistency is reached.

2. Add the mixture to popsicle molds. Tap the popsicle molds against the counter firmly to get rid of any bubbles that might have formed.
3. Press wooden spoons about two-thirds of the way into the mixture.
4. Freeze for at least five hours.
5. To unmold the popsicles, run warm water on the outside of the mold and tug the popsicle out gentle by holding onto the wooden stick.

Simple Apple Cookies

This recipes literally takes two minutes and is packed with nutrition that is good for your gut health and that gets you up and moving.

Nutritional Information

Calcium	8mg
Dietary Fiber	4g
Iron	1mg
Potassium	172mg
Protein	4g
Sodium	65mg
Sugar	10g
Total Carbohydrates	23g
Total Fat	8g
Calories per	170

serving	

Time: 2 minutes

Serving Size: 2

Ingredients:

- 1 large green apple
- 1 tablespoon of peanut butter
- 1 tablespoon of raisin

Directions:

1. Core the apple to remove the seeds. Slice the apple into round pieces.
2. Spread peanut butter on one side of each apple slice.
3. Top with raisins and eat immediately.

Tofu Nuggets

If love chicken nuggets, then you should definitely give this recipe a try!

Nutritional Information

Dietary Fiber	2.7g
Protein	12g
Sodium	184mg
Sugar	2.2g

Total Carbohydrates	20g
Total Fat	6g
Calories per serving	172

Time: 2 minutes

Serving Size: 4 (12 nuggets)

Ingredients:

- 12 pieces of ¼" thick extra firm tofu
- Olive oil
- ½ cup of soy milk
- ⅔ cup of cornmeal
- ½ teaspoon garlic powder
- ½ teaspoons of onion powder
- 1.4 teaspoon of salt

Directions:

1. Preheat your oven to 375 degrees F.
2. Prepare a baking sheet by lightly brushing it with olive oil.
3. Press the tofu pieces between paper towel to remove any extra moisture.
4. In a small bowl, mix the cornmeal, garlic powder, onion powder, and salt.
5. In another small bowl, add the milk.
6. First, dip each tofu square into the milk then the cornmeal mixture. Transfer to the coated squares to the prepared baking sheet.
7. Bake for 20 minutes on one side then flip to bake for another 15 minutes

8. Cool and serve with a condiment.

Chocolate Almond Granola Bars

Nutritional Information

Cholesterol	14mg
Dietary Fiber	5g
Protein	12g
Potassium	98mg
Sodium	327mg
Sugar	10g
Total Carbohydrates	27g
Total Fat	12g
Calories per serving	255

Time: 30 minutes

Serving Size: 8

Ingredients:

- ½ cup of vanilla protein powder
- 1 tablespoon of chia seeds
- 1 ¾ cups of oats
- 1 teaspoon of cinnamon
- ½ cup of peanut butter
- ¼ cup of maple syrup

- 2 tablespoons of mini dark chocolate chips
- 1 tablespoon of dark cocoa powder
- ½ cup of almond milk
- 2 tablespoons of chopped almonds
- A pinch of salt

Directions:

1. Preheat your oven to 350 degrees F.
2. Prepare a baking sheet with parchment paper.
3. Combine the protein powder, cocoa powder, chia seeds, oats, cinnamon, and salt in a medium bowl and mix well.
4. Microwave peanut butter and maple syrup in a small bowl for 30 seconds. Stir to mix well. Add the peanut butter mixture to the oats mixture.
5. Add the almond milk and stir into a dough.
6. Add the mixture to the baking sheet. Press the almond pieces into the dough.
7. Bake for 17 minutes.
8. Remove the tray from the oven and press the chocolate chips on top and sprinkle with the salt.
9. Let cool then cut into eight bars. Refrigerate the bars until you are ready to indulge. These can be stored in an airtight container for up to a week.

No-Bake Peanut Butter Protein Bars

Nutritional Information

Cholesterol	1mg

Dietary Fiber	2.8g
Protein	11.9g
Potassium	98mg
Sodium	14mg
Sugar	15.9g
Total Carbohydrates	29.2g
Total Fat	13.7g
Calories per serving	278

Time: 5 minutes

Serving Size: 10

Ingredients:

- 1 cup natural peanut butter
- 3/4 cup maple syrup
- 1 1/2 cups quick oats
- 1 cup vanilla protein powder

Directions:

1. Line a large tray with parchment paper.
2. Microwave peanut butter and maple syrup in a medium bowl for 30 seconds. Stir the mixture and microwave again for 30 seconds. Stir again.
3. mix in the rest of the ingredients until thoroughly combined.
4. Spread the mixture evenly across the prepared tray.
5. Leave uncovered and refrigerate for one hour.

6. Remove from the refrigerator and cut into 10 bars.
7. Cover and store in an airtight container for up to one week.

Roasted Carrot Sticks

Nutritional Information

Calcium	56mg
Dietary Fiber	4.9g
Protein	3g
Potassium	494mg
Sodium	255mg
Sugar	7.6g
Total Carbohydrates	28.9g
Total Fat	13.6g
Calories per serving	245

Time: 55 minutes

Serving Size: 4

Ingredients:

- 2 pounds of carrots peeled and cut into 1/4" thick stick
- 2 tablespoons of olive oil
- 1 teaspoon of dried oregano

- Salt and black pepper to taste.

Directions:

1. Preheat your oven to 425 degrees F.
2. Mix all the ingredients in a large bowl and toss so that the carrot sticks are thoroughly coated.
3. Place the carrot sticks in a single even layer on a baking tray.
4. Roast the carrot sticks for 35 minutes, flipping the sticks about halfway through so that they are golden on all sides.

Blueberry Chocolate Drops

Nutritional Information

Dietary Fiber	0.6g
Protein	0.7mg
Potassium	19mg
Sodium	12mg
Sugar	6.4g
Total Carbohydrates	8.5g
Total Fat	3.2g
Calories per serving	59

Time: 30 minutes

Serving Size: 12

Ingredients:

- 1 1/2 cup of melted dark chocolate chips
- 1 tablespoon of coconut oil
- 2 cup blueberries
- Salt, for garnish

Directions:

1. Prepare a baking sheet by lining it with parchment paper.
2. Arrange the blueberries in custers of about four on the baking sheets.
3. In a medium bowl, mix the chocolate and coconut oil.
4. Drizzle the chocolate mixture over the blueberries and sprinkle with salt.
5. Freeze for about 10 minutes and serve.

Dark Chocolate Mousse

Nutritional Information

Calcium	66mg
Dietary Fiber	15.8g
Protein	8.8g
Potassium	1131 mg
Sodium	693mg
Sugar	43.2g

Total Carbohydrates	70.8g
Total Fat	74.1g
Calories per serving	918

Time: 1 hour, 20 minutes

Serving Size: 2

Ingredients:

- 2 ripe avocados
- ½ cup of soy milk
- ¼ cup olive oil
- 1/2 cup of dark chocolate chips
- 1/4 cup maple syrup
- 3 tablespoon of dark cocoa powder
- 1 teaspoon vanilla extract
- 1/2 teaspoon salt

Directions:

1. Blend all the ingredients except for the chocolate chips in a blender until a smooth consistency is reached.
2. Transfer to serving glasses and refrigerated for between 30 minutes and an hour.
3. Top with the chocolate chips and serve.

Easy Banana Chocolate Mini Sandwiches

Nutritional Information

Calcium	66mg
Dietary Fiber	7g
Protein	10.3g
Potassium	529mg
Sodium	150mg
Sugar	22.9g
Total Carbohydrates	41.1g
Total Fat	22.4g
Calories per serving	379

Time: 45 minutes

Serving Size: 1

Ingredients:

- 1 firm ripe banana
- 1 tablespoon of peanut butter
- 1 tablespoon of almond chocolate butter (See Coconut Almond Toast With Dark Chocolate recipe)

Directions:

1. Slice the banana into pieces that are about half an inch thick.
2. Spread the peanut butter then the almond chocolate butter on each banana slice. Top with another piece of banana
3. You can eat these as is or place in the freezer

for 30 minutes then serve. These can be stored in the freezer in an airtight container for up to one week.

Chocolate Chia Snack Bars

Nutritional Information

Calcium	30mg
Dietary Fiber	5g
Protein	5g
Potassium	353mg
Sodium	48mg
Sugar	23g
Total Carbohydrates	32g
Total Fat	8.4g
Calories per serving	199

Time: 1 hour, 10 minutes

Serving Size: 1

Ingredients:

- 1 cup of raisins
- ¼ cup of peanut butter

- 1/4 cup of unsalted peanuts
- 2 tbsp unsweetened dark cocoa powder
- 1 1/2 tbsp chia seeds

Directions:

1. Prepare a baking sheet by lining it with parchment paper.
2. Add all the ingredients to a food processor and pulse until a coarse mixture is achieved.
3. Press the coarse mixture into prepared baking dish and refrigerate for one hour.
4. Slice into eight bars and serve. Can be stored in an airtight container in the refrigerator for one week.

No-Bake Cranberry Granola Bars

Nutritional Information

Dietary Fiber	3g
Protein	3g
Potassium	154mg
Sodium	1mg
Sugar	24g
Total Carbohydrates	38g

Total Fat	4g
Calories per serving	188

Time: 50 minutes

Serving Size: 10

Ingredients:

- 1 cup of pureed dates
- 1 cup of dried, sliced cranberries
- ¼ cup of peanut butter
- ¼ cup of maple syrup
- 1 ½ cups of rolled oats

Directions:

1. Prepare a baking sheet by lining it with parchment paper.
2. Add pureed dates, oats, and dried cranberries into a large bowl.
3. Place the maple syrup and peanut butter in a small bowl and microwave for 30 seconds. Stir to mix, then pour over oat mixture. Combine thoroughly.
4. Press the mixture to the baking sheet and refrigerate for 30 minutes.
5. Slice into 10 bars and serve. Can be stored in an airtight container in the refrigerator for one week.

Easy Chocolate Chip Cookies

Nutritional Information

Dietary Fiber	1.4g
Protein	5.8g
Potassium	121mg
Sodium	23mg
Sugar	4.7g
Total Carbohydrates	12.2g
Total Fat	2.8g
Calories per serving	91

Time: 20 minutes

Serving Size: 12

Ingredients:

- 2 tablespoons of peanut butter
- 1/3 cup dark chocolate chips
- 2 ripe bananas, mashed
- 1 ¼ cup of vanilla protein powder
- 1 cup of rolled oats

Directions:

1. Preheat your oven to 350 degrees F.
2. Prepare a baking sheet by lining it with parchment paper.
3. Mix all the ingredients together until just

combined then place spoonfuls onto the baking sheet.
4. Bake for 10 minutes or until the tops are firm.
5. Let the cookies cool. Serve.

Chapter 9: Beverages

At least 70% of the human body is made up of water. To continue to survive, the human body depends on a continuous supply to ensure that every cell, tissue, and muscle in the body continues to work at optimal conditions. Water is used to:

- Maintain the body temperature.
- Increase energy levels is especially essential before during and after exercise not only one of fatigue but to improve endurance.
- Lubricate your joints to help prevent joint diseases such as rheumatoid arthritis.
- Protect against the development of kidney stones, urinary tract infections, and constipation.
- Promotes a clear skin complexion.
- Remove waste antioxidants from the body.
- Improve the function of the brain and elevates the mood.

Drinking an adequate supply of water can even help you lose weight!

With our busy lives, we easily forget to nourish our bodies with fluids. By doing this, we risk becoming dehydrated. Signs of dehydration include low blood pressure, weakness, confusion, dry mouth, headache, extreme thirst, urine that is dark in color and no tears when crying.

It is vital that we never allow ourselves to get to the point of dehydration. We should be especially vigilant if we live in a hot climate, are sick with vomiting or diarrhea or a fever, are pregnant or breastfeeding, have medical conditions like a bladder infection or trying to lose weight.

To ward off dehydration, it is recommended that adults drink between six and eight glasses of water everyday, with eight ounces per glass! This figure however varies from individual to individual for reasons such as level of activity, weight, and height.

As clear as the need for water is in general health and wellness, it also vital to remain hydrated to prevent the trigger of inflammation.

Hydration and Chronic Inflammation

By keeping ourselves sufficiently hydrated, we are aiding the anti inflammatory process by giving the immune system the much-needed fluid it needs to keep performing at optimal conditions and to suppress proinflammatory agents such as CRP.

Some people do not like the taste of water, find it boring on the palate or otherwise have a difficult time bringing themselves to drink it. While water is the best substance for keeping hydrated, you can get your fluid intake by drinking other beverages. Teas and juices are a great way to supplement your fluid intake and you can find some of these recipes below.

Beverage Recipes

Citrus Flavored Water

Nutritional Information

Calcium	58mg
Dietary Fiber	3.2g
Protein	1.7g
Potassium	291mg
Sodium	17mg
Sugar	10.8g
Total Carbohydrates	17.8g
Total Fat	0.4g
Calories per serving	66

Time: 20 minutes

Serving Size: 4

Ingredients:

- 1 cup of sliced lemons
- ½ cup of sliced limes
- 1 cup of sliced oranges
- 2 cups of diced watermelon
- 1 cup of sliced cucumbers
- A pitcher of cold water

Directions:

1. Add all the fruit to the pitcher of water.
2. Stir well to incorporate the flavors.
3. Refrigerate the mixture for several hours before serving.

Basil-Infused Tomato Water

Nutritional Information

Calcium	27mg
Dietary Fiber	0.3g
Protein	0.3g
Potassium	9mg
Sodium	69mg
Sugar	0.7g
Total Carbohydrates	1.3g
Calories per serving	7

Time: 5 minutes

Serving Size: 4

Ingredients:

- 1 diced red tomato
- 3 branches of crushed basil
- A pitcher of cold water

Directions:

1. Add the tomato and basil to the pitcher of water.
2. Stir well to incorporate the flavors.
3. Refrigerated for at least two hours to allow the fruit flavor to infuse the water. Strain and serve chilled. This can be refrigerated up to two days.

Refreshing Strawberry Water

Nutritional Information

Calcium	16mg
Dietary Fiber	0.6g
Protein	0.3g
Potassium	65mg
Sodium	10mg
Sugar	1.5g
Total Carbohydrates	2.5g
Total Fat	0.1g

Calories per serving	10

Time: 5 minutes

Serving Size: 6

Ingredients:

- 1 cup stemmed and sliced strawberries
- 1 cup of sliced cucumbers
- A pitcher of cold water

Directions:

1. Add all the fruit to the pitcher of water.
2. Stir well to incorporate the flavors.
3. Refrigerated for at least two hours to allow the fruit flavor to infuse the water. Strain and serve chilled. This can be refrigerated up to two days.

Grapefruit Water

Nutritional Information

Calcium	14mg
Dietary Fiber	0.4g
Protein	0.2g
Potassium	56mg
Sodium	9mg
Sugar	2.7g

Total Carbohydrates	3.1g
Calories per serving	12

Time: 5 minutes

Serving Size: 6

Ingredients:

- 1 cup of fresh squeezed grapefruit juice
- A pitcher of cold water

Directions:

1. Add the grapefruit juice to the water.
2. Refrigerate and serve chilled.

Black Lemon Iced Tea

Nutritional Information

Calcium	12mg
Dietary Fiber	0.2mg
Protein	0.2g
Potassium	44mg
Sodium	10mg
Sugar	1.1g
Total Carbohydrates	1.4g
Total Fat	0.1g

Calories per serving	8

Time: 5 minutes

Serving Size: 6

Ingredients:

- 6 cups water
- 3 black tea bags
- ½ cup of stevia
- ¼ cup orange juice
- ¼ cup lemon juice
- Fresh mint leaves

Directions:

1. Bring three cups of water to a boil over medium heat in a large saucepan. Remove from the heat and steep the tea bag for five minutes.
2. Remove the tea bags and discard.
3. Move the tea to a large pitcher and add the remaining ingredients.
4. Refrigerate and served chilled. Garnish with mint.

Raspberries Iced Tea

Nutritional Information

Calcium	17mg
Dietary Fiber	3.1g

Protein	0.6g
Potassium	78mg
Sodium	23mg
Sugar	2g
Total Carbohydrates	6.1g
Total Fat	0.3g
Calories per serving	24

Time: 15 minutes

Serving Size: 8

Ingredients:

- 3 cups fresh raspberries
- ¼ cup of stevia
- 1 tablespoon chopped fresh mint
- A pinch of baking soda
- 4 cups boiling water
- 2 green tea bags

Directions:

1. Combine raspberries and stevia in large bowl. Crush the mixture with wooden spoon.
2. Add the mint and baking soda. mix and set aside.
3. Steep the tea bags in boiling water. cover and let stand three minutes then remove and Discard the tea bags.
4. Pour green tea over raspberry mixture and let

stand at room temperature for at least an hour. Strain the raspberry tea and served chilled.

Chamomile Orange Iced Tea

Nutritional Information

Calcium	11mg
Dietary Fiber	0.1g
Protein	0.2g
Potassium	91mg
Sodium	11mg
Sugar	2.6g
Total Carbohydrates	4.2g
Total Fat	0.1g
Calories per serving	14

Time: 10 minutes

Serving Size: 8

Ingredients:

- 8 chamomile tea bags
- 12 cups of boiling water
- 1 cup of orange juice
- 4 teaspoons stevia

Directions:

1. Steep the tea bags in boiling water for five minutes.
2. Remove and discard the tea back and allow the tea to cool completely before adding the remaining ingredients. Stir to mix.
3. Refrigerate and serve chilled or with ice.

Mint Tea

Nutritional Information

Calcium	12mg
Dietary Fiber	0.2g
Protein	0.1g
Potassium	19mg
Sodium	8mg
Total Carbohydrates	1g
Calories per serving	1

Time: 10 minutes

Serving Size: 5

Ingredients:

- 5 cups of boiling water
- 2 green tea bags
- 6 mint leaves
- 4 teaspoons stevia

Directions:

1. Steep the tea bags in boiling water for five minutes.
2. Remove and discard the tea back and allow the tea to cool completely before adding the remaining ingredients. Stir to mix.
3. Strain and serve immediately. This can be refrigerated and served chilled.

Basil Ginger Tea

Nutritional Information

Calcium	36mg
Dietary Fiber	0.1g
Protein	0.2g
Potassium	27mg
Sodium	29mg
Total Carbohydrates	0.4g
Total Fat	0.1g
Calories per serving	2

Time: 15 minutes

Serving Size: 2

Ingredients:

- 3 large basil leaves

- ½ teaspoon of finely grated ginger
- Boiled water

Directions:

1. Add all the ingredients to a teapot and brew until it reached your desired strength.
2. Sieve the basil and ginger, and serve
3. This beverage can be served cold by adding ice or refrigerating.

Green Veggie Juice

This juice is packed with ingredients that fight chronic inflammation while strengthening the body's natural defenses. In particular, the pineapple in this recipe, is high in a compound called bromelain which is suppressing proinflammatory indicators. It is particularly great for people who suffer from arthritis symptoms. And the biggest benefit? It is absolutely delicious.

Nutritional Information

Calcium	66mg
Dietary Fiber	5.5g
Folate	32mg
Vitamin A	1512µg
Vitamin C	27mg
Vitamin K	81mg
Iron	1.3mg
Magnesium	12.5mg

Potassium	532mg
Zinc	0.2mg
Protein	2g
Sugars	16g
Total Carbohydrates	28g
Total Fat	0g
Calories per serving	114

Time: 5 minutes

Serving Size: 2

Ingredients:

- 4 celery stalks
- ½ cup of diced cucumber
- 1 cup of diced pineapple
- ½ cup of diced green apple
- 1 cup of washed spinach
- 1 lemon
- ¼ cup of sliced ginger

Directions:

1. Add all the ingredients to a juicer and juice.
2. Consume the juice immediately.

Pineapple Juice

Nutritional Information

Calcium	27mg
Dietary Fiber	2.4g
Protein	1g
Potassium	199mg
Sodium	689mg
Sugar	16.4g
Total Carbohydrates	22.2g
Total Fat	0.1g
Calories per serving	86

Time: 10 minutes

Serving Size: 2

Ingredients:

- 2 cups of cubed pineapple
- 1 cup of water
- ½ inch of ginger
- ½ teaspoon of salt
- 3 basil leaves
- 1 tablespoon of lemon juice

Directions:

1. Add all the ingredients to a blender and blend

until smooth.
2. Strain to remove solid bit and serve immediately. Can be served with ice.

Mango Juice

Nutritional Information

Calcium	14mg
Dietary Fiber	1.1g
Protein	1.3g
Potassium	334mg
Sodium	4mg
Sugar	16g
Total Carbohydrates	19.5g
Total Fat	0.1g
Calories per serving	83

Time: 10 minutes

Serving Size: 4

Ingredients:

- 1 cups of cubed ripe mango
- 2 cup of orange juice
- 1 cup of water
- ½ inch of ginger
- 5 mint leaves

Directions:

1. Add all the ingredients to a blender and blend until smooth.
2. Serve immediately. Can be served with ice.

Cucumber Celery Juice

Nutritional Information

Dietary Fiber	1.3g
Protein	0.4g
Potassium	85mg
Sodium	60mg
Sugar	1.9g
Total Carbohydrates	4.2g
Total Fat	0.1g
Calories per serving	19

Time: 5 minutes

Serving Size: 2

Ingredients:

- 2 cups of cubed cucumber
- 2 cups of sliced celery sticks
- 1 cup of ice cubes
- 1 cup of water
- ½ inch of ginger

- Salt and black pepper to taste

Directions:

1. Add all the ingredients to a blender and blend until smooth.
2. Serve immediately.

Detoxifying Fruit Juice

Nutritional Information

Dietary Fiber	3.8g
Protein	1.3g
Potassium	361mg
Sodium	38mg
Sugar	13.1g
Total Carbohydrates	19.1g
Total Fat	0.5g
Calories per serving	77

Time: 5 minutes

Serving Size: 4

Ingredients:

- 2 cups of spinach
- 1 cup sliced celery
- 2 cups diced cucumber

- 2 tablespoons of lemon juice
- 2 cups diced red Apples
- 1-2 inch ginger
- 1 cup of water

Directions:

1. Add all the ingredients to a blender and blend until smooth.
2. Serve immediately. Can be served with ice.

Creamy Chai Tea

This tea is flavorful and gives you the boost you need to have a productive day. In addition, the ingredient cardamom is known for improving blood circulation, while cinnamon helps regulate blood sugar and boosts immunity.

Nutritional Information

Dietary Fiber	2g
Cholesterol	1mg
Vitamin A	1010µg
Vitamin C	12mg
Iron	1.4mg
Protein	1g
Sugars	2g
Total Carbohydrates	6g
Total Fat	1g

Calories per serving	29

Time: 10 minutes

Serving Size: 3

Ingredients:

- 1 ¼ cup of water
- ½ cup of soymilk
- 1 ½ teaspoon stevia
- 2 crushed cloves
- 1 stick of cinnamon
- 2 crushed cardamom pods
- 1 ½ tablespoons black tea leaves

Directions:

1. Bring the water and all the spices to a boil. Cover the pot and simmer for three minutes.
2. Add the milk and stevia. Stir and allow the mixture to come to a gentle boil
3. Take off the heat and add the black tea leaves. Steep the leaves for five minutes.
4. Sieves the tea to remove the leaves and spices.
5. Serve warm.

Spiced Hot Chocolate

When most people think hot chocolate, they think of Christmas, but this recipe is great all year round. It is loaded with spices and all the great anti inflammation benefits.

Nutritional Information

Dietary Fiber	2.3g
Potassium	173mg
Vitamin D	1mcg
Iron	2mg
Protein	1g
Sugars	0.7g
Total Carbohydrates	6.6g
Total Fat	0.1g
Calories per serving	46

Time: 10 minutes

Serving Size: 2

Ingredients:

- 2 cups unsweetened cashew milk
- 2 tablespoons of dark cocoa or cacao powder
- 2 tablespoon pumpkin purée
- ⅛ teaspoon ground cinnamon
- A pinch of ground nutmeg
- A pinch of ground ginger
- ⅛ tsp liquid stevia

Directions:

1. Add all the ingredients to a small pan and whisk as it comes to a boil over medium heat. This should take less than three minutes.
2. Pour into two cups and serve immediately.

Conclusion

Chronic inflammation does not have to control your life any longer and best of all you do not have to make dramatic changes to ensure it does not. All it takes is awareness and simple changes to your lifestyle to you diet so that you live happier, healthier, and pain free. Living with chronic inflammation can make life seem hopeless and dreary. This book aims at being your light at the end of the tunnel. There is a lot of misinformation out there about chronic inflammation its cause and its preventive measures. This book, which is based on sound research and proven scientific principles, cuts through the clutter and gets straight to the heart of the matter. The recipes detailed are aimed at not only helping you fight chronic inflammation, but also at helping you achieve generally good health all around in addition to being delicious. You have reached the end of this book and I congratulate you on being dedicated to improving your health and your life. It is indeed a huge step in gaining the knowledge that you need to fight this disease.

The next step is to put what you have learned into practice. Luckily, that action partly involves putting your culinary skills to good use, something that can be quite fun.

Thank you for downloading this book! I wish you success in taking control of your life and finally defeating chronic inflammation.

Finally, if you found this book useful in any way, a review on Amazon is always appreciated!

References

Aloysius T. A., Carvajal A. K., Slizyte R., Skorve J., Berge R. K., Bjørndal B. (2018). Chicken Protein Hydrolysates Have Anti-Inflammatory Effects on High-Fat Diet Induced Obesity in Mice. *Medicines (Basel)*. 6(1). pii: E5. doi: 10.3390/medicines6010005.

Avena, N. M., Rada, P., & Hoebel, B. G. (2008). Evidence for sugar addiction: behavioral and neurochemical effects of intermittent, excessive sugar intake. *Neuroscience and biobehavioral reviews*, 32(1), 20–39. doi:10.1016/j.neubiorev.2007.04.019

Bawaked, R. A., Schröder, H., Ribas-Barba, L., Izquierdo-Pulido, M., Pérez-Rodrigo, C., Fíto, M., & Serra-Majem, L. (2017). Association of diet quality with dietary inflammatory potential in youth. *Food & nutrition research*, 61(1), 1328961. doi:10.1080/16546628.2017.1328961

Bosma-den Boer, M. M., van Wetten, M. L., & Pruimboom, L. (2012). Chronic inflammatory diseases are stimulated by current lifestyle: how diet, stress levels and medication prevent our body from recovering. *Nutrition & metabolism*, 9(1), 32. doi:10.1186/1743-7075-9-32

Calder P. C. (2010). Omega-3 fatty acids and inflammatory processes. *Nutrients*, 2(3), 355–374. doi:10.3390/nu2030355

Chacko, S. M., Thambi, P. T., Kuttan, R., & Nishigaki, I. (2010). Beneficial effects of green tea: a literature review.

Chinese medicine, 5, 13. doi:10.1186/1749-8546-5-13

Chai, W., Morimoto, Y., Cooney, R. V., Franke, A. A., Shvetsov, Y. B., Le Marchand, L., ... Maskarinec, G. (2017). Dietary Red and Processed Meat Intake and Markers of Adiposity and Inflammation: *The Multiethnic Cohort Study. Journal of the American College of Nutrition, 36*(5), 378-385. doi:10.1080/07315724.2017.1318317

Chatterjee, P., Chandra, S., Dey, P., & Bhattacharya, S. (2012). Evaluation of anti-inflammatory effects of green tea and black tea: A comparative in vitro study. *Journal of advanced pharmaceutical technology & research, 3*(2), 136-138. doi:10.4103/2231-4040.97298

Chen, L., Deng, H., Cui, H., Fang, J., Zuo, Z., Deng, J., ... Zhao, L. (2017). Inflammatory responses and inflammation-associated diseases in organs. *Oncotarget, 9*(6), 7204-7218. doi:10.18632/oncotarget.23208

Della Corte, K. W., Perrar, I., Penczynski, K. J., Schwingshackl, L., Herder, C., & Buyken, A. E. (2018). Effect of Dietary Sugar Intake on Biomarkers of Subclinical Inflammation: A Systematic Review and Meta-Analysis of Intervention Studies. *Nutrients, 10*(5), 606. doi:10.3390/nu10050606

Ellulu, M. S., Rahmat, A., Patimah, I., Khaza'ai, H., & Abed, Y. (2015). Effect of vitamin C on inflammation and metabolic markers in hypertensive and/or diabetic obese adults: a randomized controlled trial. *Drug design, development and therapy, 9*, 3405-3412. doi:10.2147/DDDT.S83144

Gao, Y., Bielohuby, M., Fleming, T., Grabner, G. F., Foppen, E., Bernhard, W., ... Yi, C. X. (2017). Dietary sugars, not lipids, drive hypothalamic inflammation. *Molecular metabolism, 6(8),* 897–908. doi:10.1016/j.molmet.2017.06.008

Grieger, J. A., Miller, M. D., & Cobiac, L. (2014). Investigation of the effects of a high fish diet on inflammatory cytokines, blood pressure, and lipids in healthy older Australians. *Food & nutrition research, 58,* 10.3402/fnr.v58.20369. doi:10.3402/fnr.v58.20369

Kiecolt-Glaser J. K. (2010). Stress, food, and inflammation: psychoneuroimmunology and nutrition at the cutting edge. *Psychosomatic medicine, 72(4),* 365–369. doi:10.1097/PSY.0b013e3181dbf489

Kim M. E., Na J. Y., Park Y. D., Lee J. S. (2018). Anti-Neuroinflammatory Effects of Vanillin Through the Regulation of Inflammatory Factors and NF-κB Signaling in LPS-Stimulated Microglia. *Appl Biochem Biotechnol.* 187(3):884-893. doi: 10.1007/s12010-018-2857-5

Khanna, S., Jaiswal, K. S., & Gupta, B. (2017). Managing Rheumatoid Arthritis with Dietary Interventions. *Frontiers in nutrition, 4,* 52. doi:10.3389/fnut.2017.00052

Kunnumakkara, A. B., Sailo, B. L., Banik, K., Harsha, C., Prasad, S., Gupta, S. C., ... Aggarwal, B. B. (2018). Chronic diseases, inflammation, and spices: how are they linked?. *Journal of translational medicine, 16(1),* 14. doi:10.1186/s12967-018-1381-2

Lawrence, T., & Gilroy, D. W. (2007). Chronic inflammation: a failure of resolution?. *International journal of experimental pathology, 88(2),* 85–94. doi:10.1111/j.1365-2613.2006.00507.x

Liu, Y. Z., Wang, Y. X., & Jiang, C. L. (2017). Inflammation:

The Common Pathway of Stress-Related Diseases. *Frontiers in human neuroscience, 11,* 316. doi:10.3389/fnhum.2017.00316

Martins, G. R., Gelaleti, G. B., Moschetta, M. G., Maschio-Signorini, L. B., & Zuccari, D. A. (2016). Proinflammatory and Anti-Inflammatory Cytokines Mediated by NF-κB Factor as Prognostic Markers in Mammary Tumors. *Mediators of inflammation, 2016,* 9512743. doi:10.1155/2016/9512743

Mashhadi, N. S., Ghiasvand, R., Askari, G., Hariri, M., Darvishi, L., & Mofid, M. R. (2013). Anti-oxidative and anti-inflammatory effects of ginger in health and physical activity: review of current evidence. *International journal of preventive medicine, 4*(Suppl 1), S36–S42.

Minihane, A. M., Vinoy, S., Russell, W. R., Baka, A., Roche, H. M., Tuohy, K. M., ... Calder, P. C. (2015). Low-grade inflammation, diet composition and health: current research evidence and its translation. *The British journal of nutrition, 114*(7), 999–1012. doi:10.1017/S0007114515002093

Mullington, J. M., Simpson, N. S., Meier-Ewert, H. K., & Haack, M. (2010). Sleep loss and inflammation. *Best practice & research. Clinical endocrinology & metabolism, 24*(5), 775–784. doi:10.1016/j.beem.2010.08.014

Na, W., Kim, M., & Sohn, C. (2018). Dietary inflammatory index and its relationship with high-sensitivity C-reactive protein in Korean: data from the health examinee cohort. *Journal of clinical biochemistry and nutrition, 62*(1), 83–88. doi:10.3164/jcbn.17-22

Punchard, N. A., Whelan, C. J., & Adcock, I. (2004). *The*

Journal of Inflammation. *Journal of inflammation (London, England), 1*(1), 1. doi:10.1186/1476-9255-1-1

Sears, B., & Ricordi, C. (2011). Anti-inflammatory nutrition as a pharmacological approach to treat obesity. *Journal of obesity, 2011*, 431985. doi:10.1155/2011/431985

Shivappa, N., Hebert, J. R., Neshatbini Tehrani, A., Bayzai, B., Naja, F., & Rashidkhani, B. (2018). A Pro-Inflammatory Diet Is Associated With an Increased Odds of Depression Symptoms Among Iranian Female Adolescents: A Cross-Sectional Study. *Frontiers in psychiatry, 9*, 400. doi:10.3389/fpsyt.2018.00400

Straub, R. H., & Schradin, C. (2016). Chronic inflammatory systemic diseases: An evolutionary trade-off between acutely beneficial but chronically harmful programs. *Evolution, medicine, and public health, 2016*(1), 37–51. doi:10.1093/emph/eow001

Thring, T. S., Hili, P., & Naughton, D. P. (2011). Antioxidant and potential anti-inflammatory activity of extracts and formulations of white tea, rose, and witch hazel on primary human dermal fibroblast cells. *Journal of inflammation (London, England), 8*(1), 27. doi:10.1186/1476-9255-8-27

Turner, K. M., Keogh, J. B., Meikle, P. J., & Clifton, P. M. (2017). Changes in Lipids and Inflammatory Markers after Consuming Diets High in Red Meat or Dairy for Four Weeks. *Nutrients, 9*(8), 886. doi:10.3390/nu9080886

Westwater, M. L., Fletcher, P. C., & Ziauddeen, H. (2016). Sugar addiction: the state of the science. *European journal of nutrition, 55*(Suppl 2), 55–69. doi:10.1007/s00394-016-1229-6

Wiss, D. A., Avena, N., & Rada, P. (2018). Sugar Addiction: From Evolution to Revolution. *Frontiers in psychiatry, 9*, 545. doi:10.3389/fpsyt.2018.00545

Wojdasiewicz, P., Poniatowski, Ł. A., & Szukiewicz, D. (2014). The role of inflammatory and anti-inflammatory cytokines in the pathogenesis of osteoarthritis. *Mediators of inflammation, 2014*, 561459. doi:10.1155/2014/561459

Woods, J. A., Wilund, K. R., Martin, S. A., & Kistler, B. M. (2012). Exercise, inflammation and aging. *Aging and disease,* 3(1), 130–140.

Xin, W., Wei, W., & Li, X. (2012). Effects of fish oil supplementation on inflammatory markers in chronic heart failure: a meta-analysis of randomized controlled trials. *BMC cardiovascular disorders, 12*, 77. doi:10.1186/1471-2261-12-77

Zhang, J. M., & An, J. (2007). Cytokines, inflammation, and pain. *International anesthesiology clinics,* 45(2), 27–37. doi:10.1097/AIA.0b013e318034194e

www.ingramcontent.com/pod-product-compliance
Lightning Source LLC
Chambersburg PA
CBHW070621220526
45466CB00001B/71